Mouth Madness
Oral Motor Activities for Children

Catherine Orr, M.A., OTR, BCP

Illustrations by Nora Voutas

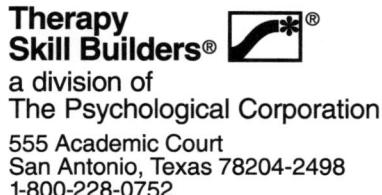

a division of
The Psychological Corporation

555 Academic Court
San Antonio, Texas 78204-2498
1-800-228-0752

Copyright © 1998 by

**Therapy
Skill Builders®**
a division of
The Psychological Corporation

555 Academic Court
San Antonio, Texas 78204-2498
1-800-228-0752

All rights reserved. No part of this publication may be reproduced or transmitted in any form or by any means, electronic or mechanical, including photocopy, recording, or any information storage and retrieval system, without permission in writing from the publisher.

The *Learning Curve Design* and *Therapy Skill Builders* are registered trademarks of The Psychological Corporation.

076164850X

9 10 11 12 A B C D E

Printed in the United States of America.

Visit our website at www.hbtpc.com.

This book is dedicated to the adults and the children at Callier Preschool for the joy in life and learning that flows from their work together.

A special thanks to Kristen McNutt for her contribution to the activities, and to Melissa Mitchell for her visualization of this work.

About the Author

Catherine Orr is an occupational therapist with extensive experience in school-based settings. She is an assistant professor in the School of Occupational Therapy at Texas Woman's University. Ms. Orr also provides therapy services to the children at Callier Preschool, the regional day school for the deaf in the Dallas area.

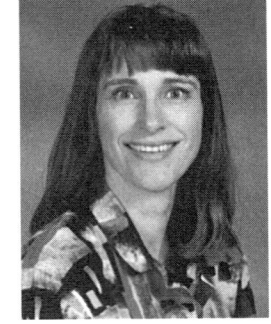

Ms. Orr received her bachelor's degree in Occupational Therapy from the University of Kansas and Master of Arts in Occupational Therapy from Texas Woman's University. She holds a specialty certification in pediatrics, is certified in the administration of the Sensory Integration and Praxis Tests, and is pursuing a doctoral degree in Kinesiology, Motor Learning and Control.

Although Ms. Orr has always had a penchant for rhymes and games, it was her experiences with the children at Callier that inspired this book.

Contents

Welcome to *Mouth Madness!* 1–2
Who Can Use the Activities? 1
What Are the Activities? 2
Oral Action Plays 2
Mouth Games 2
Silly Snacks 2
Alliteration Songs 2

Oral Action Plays 3–53
About the Oral Action Plays 5
Lips 7–26
Bellamy 8–9
Blah-Blah-Blah-Blah-Blah! 10
Brush Your Teeth 11
Fishy-Wishy 12–13
Dirt in Your Mouth 14
Flat Tire 15
The Lost Mouth 16–17
Kissy Missy, Kissy Mister 18
Peek-a-Boo Face 19–21
Driving the Car 22–23
The Sneeze 24–25
Smiles and Frowns 26
Cheeks 27–40
Balloon Blow 28–30
A Ball in Your Mouth 31
Bubba's Bubble 32
Fat Cat 33
Dirty Eyeballs 34–35
The Fly 36–37
The Worm 38–39
Toadie Fingers 40

Tongue 41–53
    The Butterflies 42
    Button Head 43
    Careful Willie 44–45
    I Can Count My Teeth 46
    The Super-Clean Worm 47
    Momma Kitty 48
    About Snakes 49
    This Little Piggy 50–51
    Stamp Licking 52
    Zip It! 53

Mouth Games 55–87
  About the Mouth Games 57–58
    Straws 57–58
  Blowing 59–74
    Blow Me Over 60
    Bottle o' Bubbles 61
    Cotton Ball Clear-Out 62
    Firefighters 63
    Glitter Blow 64
    Floating Cups 65
    Party-Favor Ball Race 66
    Pinwheels 67
    Playing-Card People 68
    Blowing Down the Road 69
    Pooh! 70
    Pucker Power 71
    Rattle Blow 72
    Visual and Kinesthetic Whistles 73
    Water Table Boats 74
  Manipulating 75–87
    Crayon Mouth Sticks 76
    Mister Chin Man 77
    Kissing Pictures 78
    Mustache Trick 79
    Muffle Face 80

    Natural Mouth Kazoos 81
        Annie's Cheek Pull 81
        Clown Grin 81
        Steel Guitar Sound Effect 81
    Puppy Pick-Up Sticks 82
    Ring Fetch 83
    It's a Tornado! 84
    Typewriter Carriage 85
    The Vacuum Cleaner 86
    Which Way Did It Go? 87

Silly Snacks 89–109
About Silly Snacks 91
    Banana Shish Kebabs 92
    Bobbing for Grapes 93
    Caramel Puffed Plates 94
    Cereal Loop Bracelets 95
    Dainty Peas 96
    Dangling Pretzels 97
    Duck's Bill Potato Chips 98
    "Everybody's Done It" Spaghetti Slurp 99
    Folding Cheese 100
    Orange-Peel Smiles 101
    Mystery Pictures 102
    Peanut Butter Cups 103
    Raisin Anteater Trail 104
    Squeeze-Cheese Trails 105
    Stacking Marshmallow Blocks 106
    Sweet Goat Nibbles 107
    Dog-Bowl Races 108
    Whipped Cream All Over 109

Alliteration Songs 111–135
About the Alliteration Songs 113
Alliteration Warm-Ups 113
    Magic Fingers 113
    Motor Boat Song 113

Songs 114–135
    Bee Bobble Bibble Bobble Boo! 114
    Chewy-Chewy Chaw 115
    Derry-Down-Nitty 116
    Fingle, Flyger, Feather Stuff 117
    Goop 118-119
    My Old Mule, Hugh 120
    Jolly Jiggles 121
    Kuh-Kuh-Kuh-Roo! 122-123
    Lulla-Baby 124-125
    Mounds of Mushy Fruit 126
    Ninny-Nanny-Noo! 127
    Purple Pipple Pop 128
    Raving and Raring to Roar! 129
    Sally, the Silly Snake 130
    Tippie-Tappie 131
    Vittles in the Vat 132
    Wiggle-Wiggle, Whompa-Whompa, Woo! 133
    Yippee! Yappie! Ki-Yi-Yay! 134
    Zap! 135

Welcome to Mouth Madness!

Mouth Madness is a book of young children's activities that emphasize mouth movements. Most activity books provide games for the hands or body. *Mouth Madness* provides games for the mouth. It fills a need for oral motor practice that is fun and motivating. *Mouth Madness* activities can supplement occupational therapy, speech therapy, or education programs where oral motor coordination and skill is a goal.

Oral motor skills are most commonly addressed within the context of feeding or speech articulation. In *Mouth Madness,* oral motor activities are presented in a game format similar to that used in training fine or gross motor development. The emphasis of the games is on directly imitating and planning new motor movements. Retention and transfer of a motor skill are enhanced by varying the conditions of practice for that skill. The activities in *Mouth Madness* are created to provide this variety for oral motor skill development and provide practice of oral motor movements.

The activities are fun, and the games have a strong motivational component. Activities may be selected to target individual problems, or the games can be used in a group situation. The activities provide a natural focus to the mouth that can be shared by classmates or friends who do not have oral motor challenges.

Who Can Use the Activities?

The activities in *Mouth Madness* are designed for children as young as three and up to age eight, with an oral motor developmental level of three years. The activities are not designed for children with severe mental or physical challenges. Children must be able to independently and effectively consume a standard meal to participate in the Silly Snacks activities.

The activities are appropriate for treatment of oral motor challenges in children with articulation or phonological disorders, dysarthria, dyspraxia, or hearing impairments where speech acquisition is a goal.

To enjoy the activities, children must have the ability to hear some speech sounds, receptive language capabilities at a minimum developmental level of 2½ years, and the ability to attend to and understand cause-effect games. Many of the activities are most effective in a small-group setting. The inclusion of peers without oral motor challenges is encouraged in these groupings.

What Are the Activities?

Mouth Madness contains activities in four sections—Oral Action Plays, Mouth Games, Silly Snacks, and Alliteration Songs. Instructions are given at the beginning of each section.

Oral Action Plays

Oral action plays are simple "finger plays" done with the mouth. Mouth movements are matched to a story or rhyme. Most of the stories contain a joke or punch line and use "funny face" mouth positions. Participation in oral action plays encourages close attention to mouth movements and their imitation. The plays are presented in three sections matching the body part—the lips, cheeks, or tongue—that is most active in the play.

Mouth Games

Mouth Games are contests and short cause-effect activities. These games require some simple materials such as table-tennis balls or empty plastic soda bottles. The games are organized by the primary action required to participate—either blowing or manipulating. Mouth games require the child to plan new motor movements in order to accomplish the game tasks.

Silly Snacks

Silly Snacks introduce funny ways to eat food. Most of the activities involve eating without using the hands, and they encourage children to move their mouths in new ways. They create a motor planning connection between eating and the new mouth movements.

Silly Snacks are not recommended for children with pronounced eating difficulties. These games are designed only for children who can independently and effectively consume a standard meal.

Foods used are typical snack foods such as loop cereal, raisins, and marshmallows. *Individual children's dietary restrictions must be followed when using these snack games.*

Alliteration Songs

Alliteration songs are based on consonant sounds. In each song, a consonant sound is combined with several vowel phonemes. The songs provide practice in making consonant sounds in varied combinations. To increase the children's interest, each alliteration song is matched with a game or an action. Alliteration songs provide varied practice in the oral movements required to create speech.

Oral Action Plays

About the Oral Action Plays

Oral action plays are simple "finger plays" done with the mouth. Conduct them in a one-on-one instructional setting, or introduce them in a small group. A group will entice interest and provide the children with more models to work from.

Lead the play by reciting a line of the rhyme or story, and then model the mouth action that corresponds to that line. Encourage the children to mimic the mouth action. Dramatic exaggeration of the action and the mouth movements helps to hold the children's attention. You may have the children recite the stories, but primarily encourage them to mimic the movements.

The oral action plays are presented in three sections—Lips, Cheeks, and Tongue. These categories refer to the mouth part that is most emphasized in the play. Exact replication of the facial movements is *not* the goal of the activities. The major benefit of playing is in learning to watch and imitate mouth movement. This benefit will be achieved more readily within an atmosphere of fun. Praise and encourage any attempt.

Lips

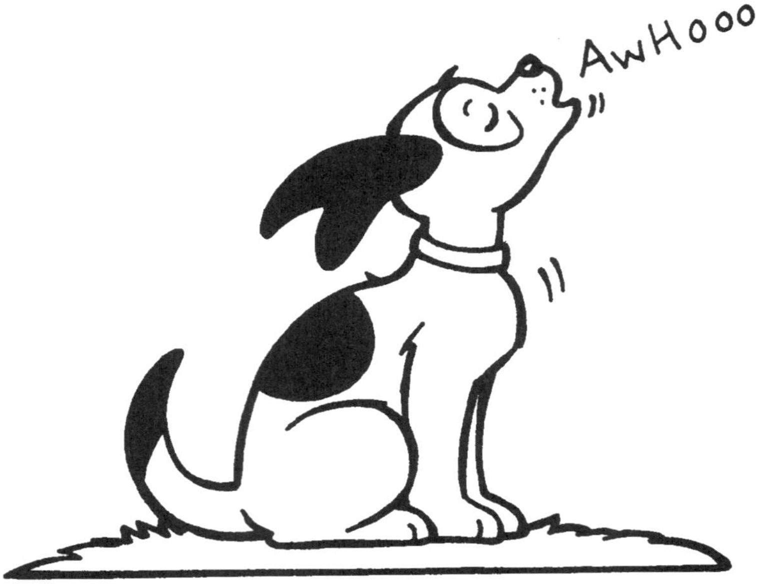

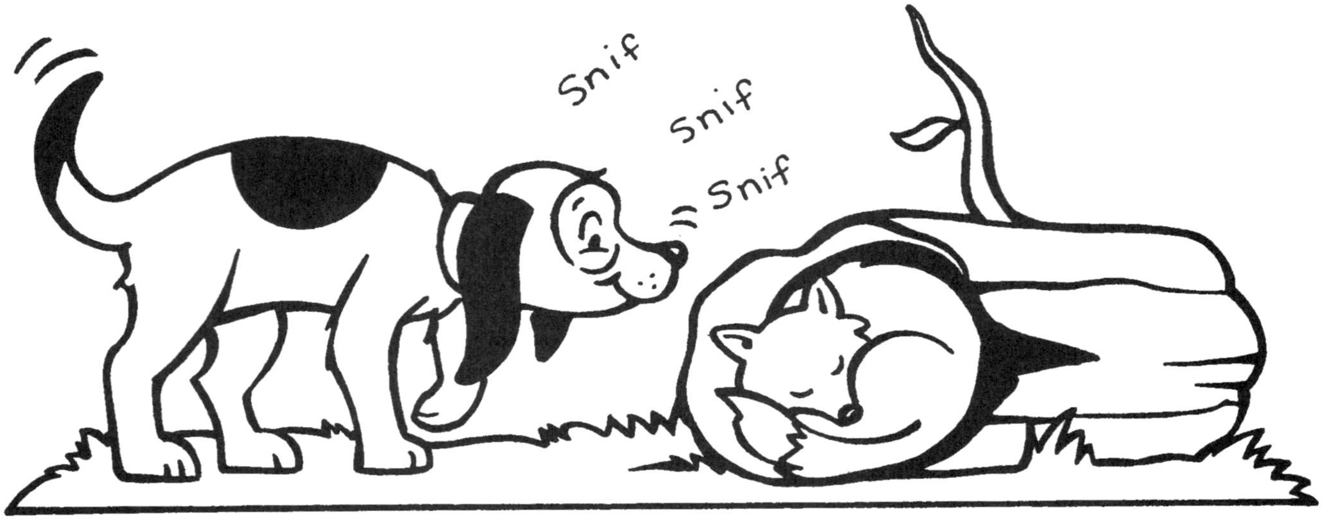

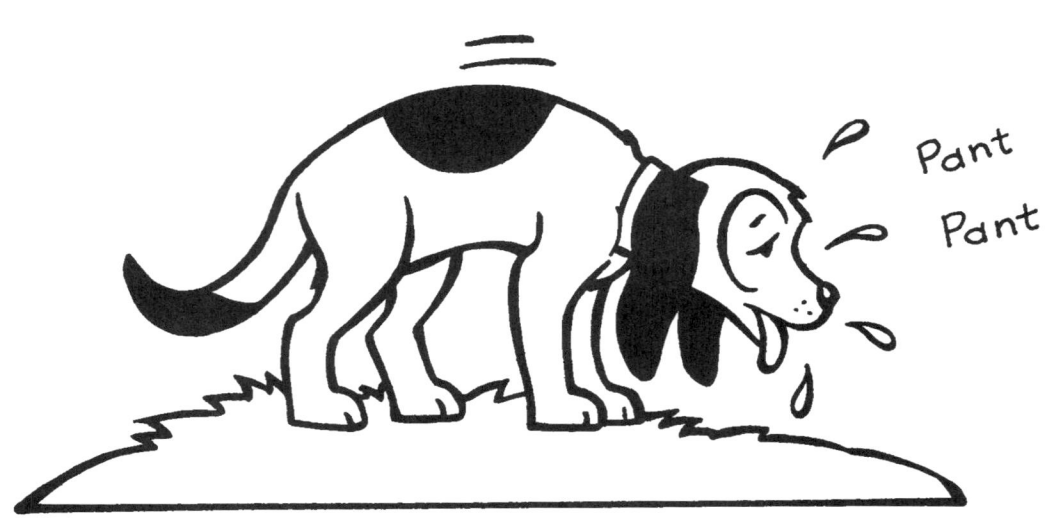

Bellamy

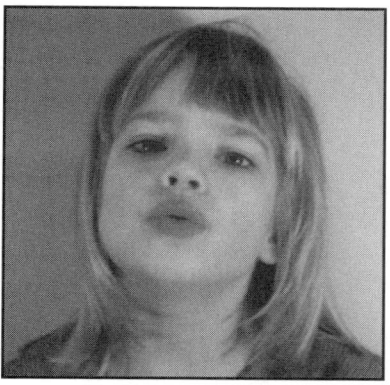

Hear Bellamy the hunting hound.
Awhoo! Awhoo!
Hear Bellamy the hunting hound.
Awhoo! Awhoo!

Make exaggerated ooo mouth shapes as Bellamy says, "Awhoo!"

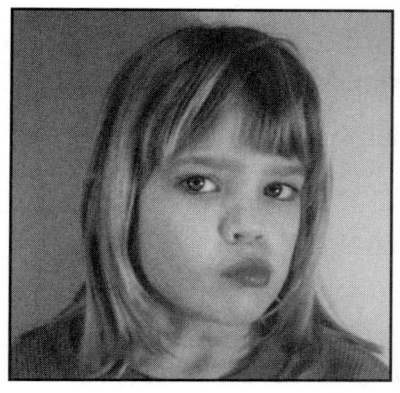 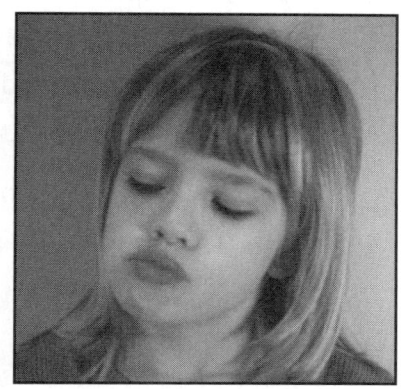

Hear Bellamy the hunting hound.
He'll catch the fox, that's true.
Watch him sniffing all around.

Pucker lips and move them to the right and left with exaggerated sniffs.

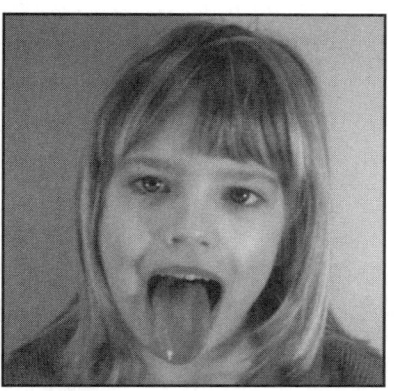

See his tongue hang to the ground.

Stick out tongue and pant.

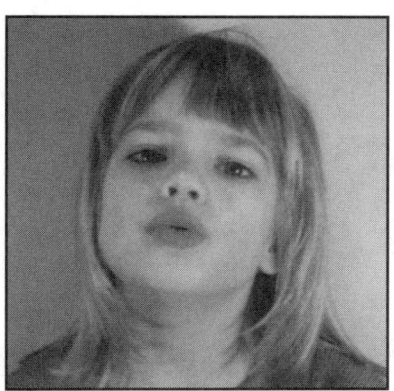

Hear Bellamy the hunting hound.
Awhoo! Awhoo!
He's the loudest sound around!

Make exaggerated ooo mouth shapes as Bellamy says, "Awhoo!"

Blah-Blah-Blah-Blah-Blah!

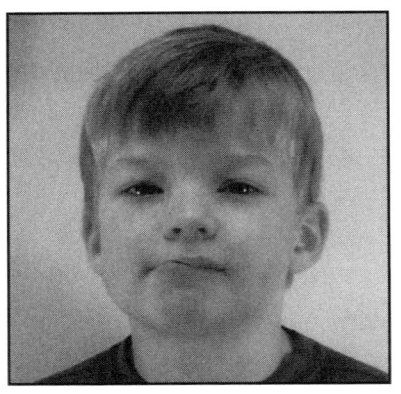

What do you do while the big people talk?
Blah-blah-blah-blah-blah!
What do you do while the big people talk?
Blah-blah-blah-blah-blah!
Lip lock, lip lock! Lock your lips!

Slide lower jaw horizontally to the right. Fold right lower lip over right upper lip.

What do you do while the big people talk?
Blah-blah-blah-blah-blah!
What do you do while the big people talk?
Blah-blah-blah-blah-blah!
Lip lock, lip lock! Lock your lips!

Reverse the action, sliding lower jaw horizontally to the left. Fold left upper lip over left lower lip.

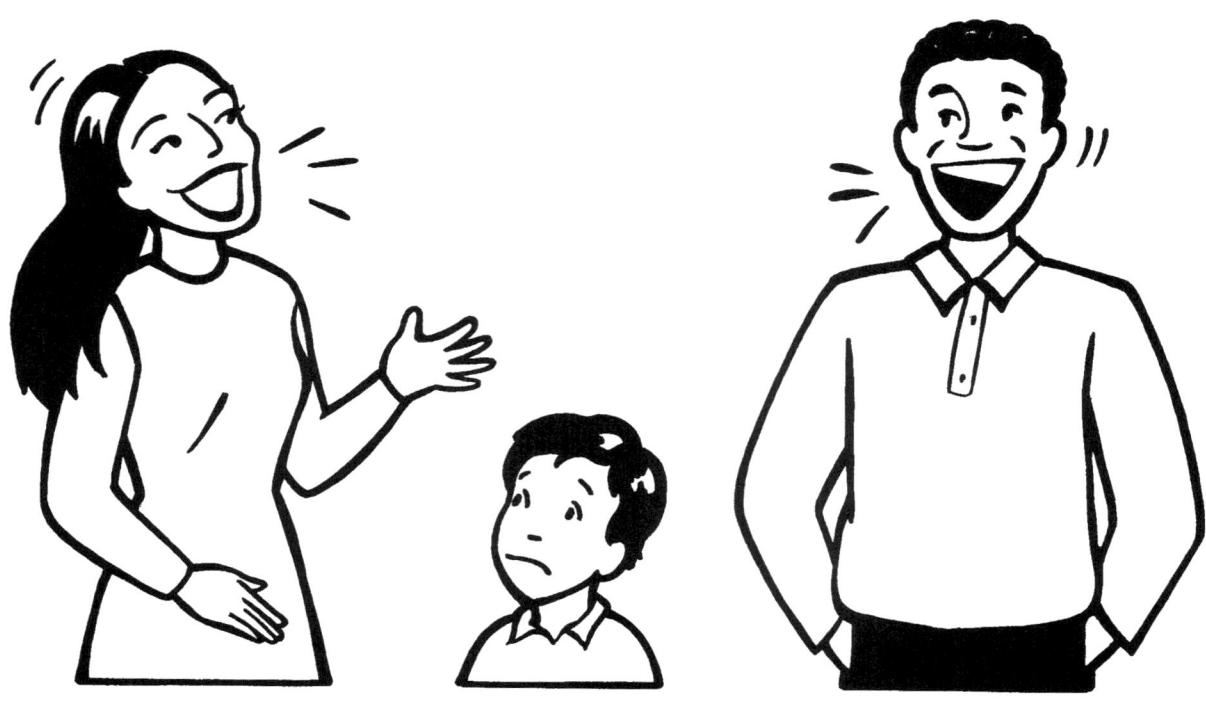

Brush Your Teeth

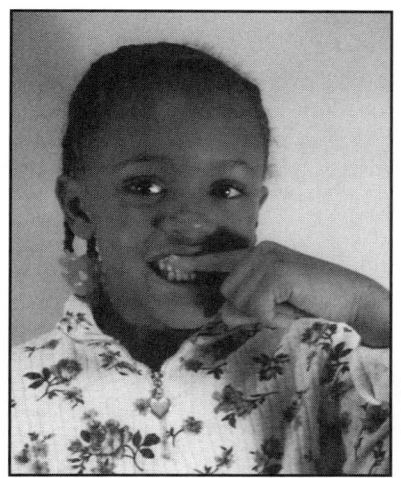

Brush your teeth every day.

Bare teeth and mime finger as toothbrush.

Brush your teeth every day.

Repeat the action.

Brush your teeth every day.

Repeat the action.

Brush them or they'll go away!

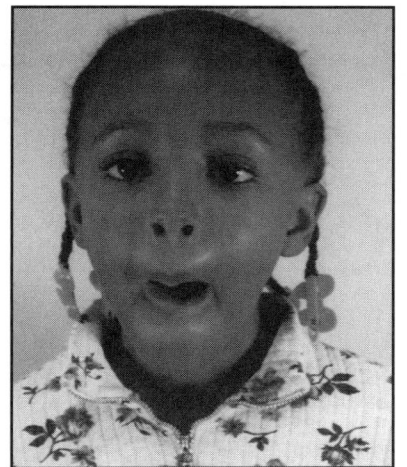

Open mouth, cover teeth with lips, and show surprise at "losing teeth."

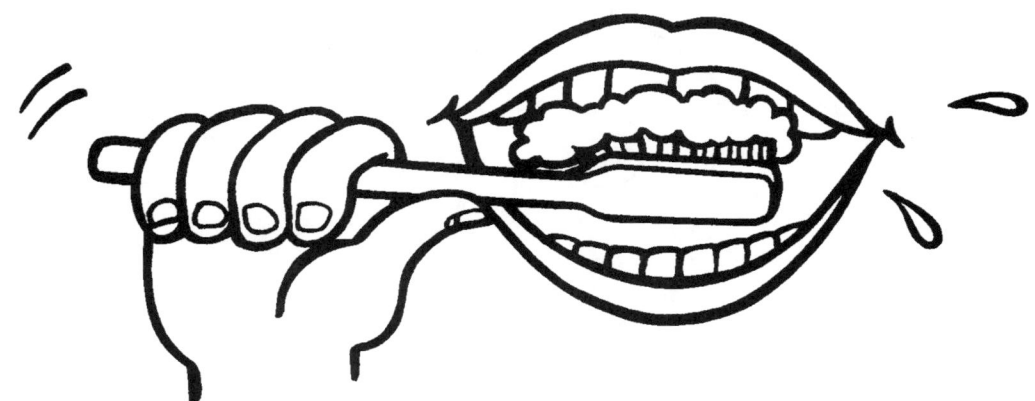

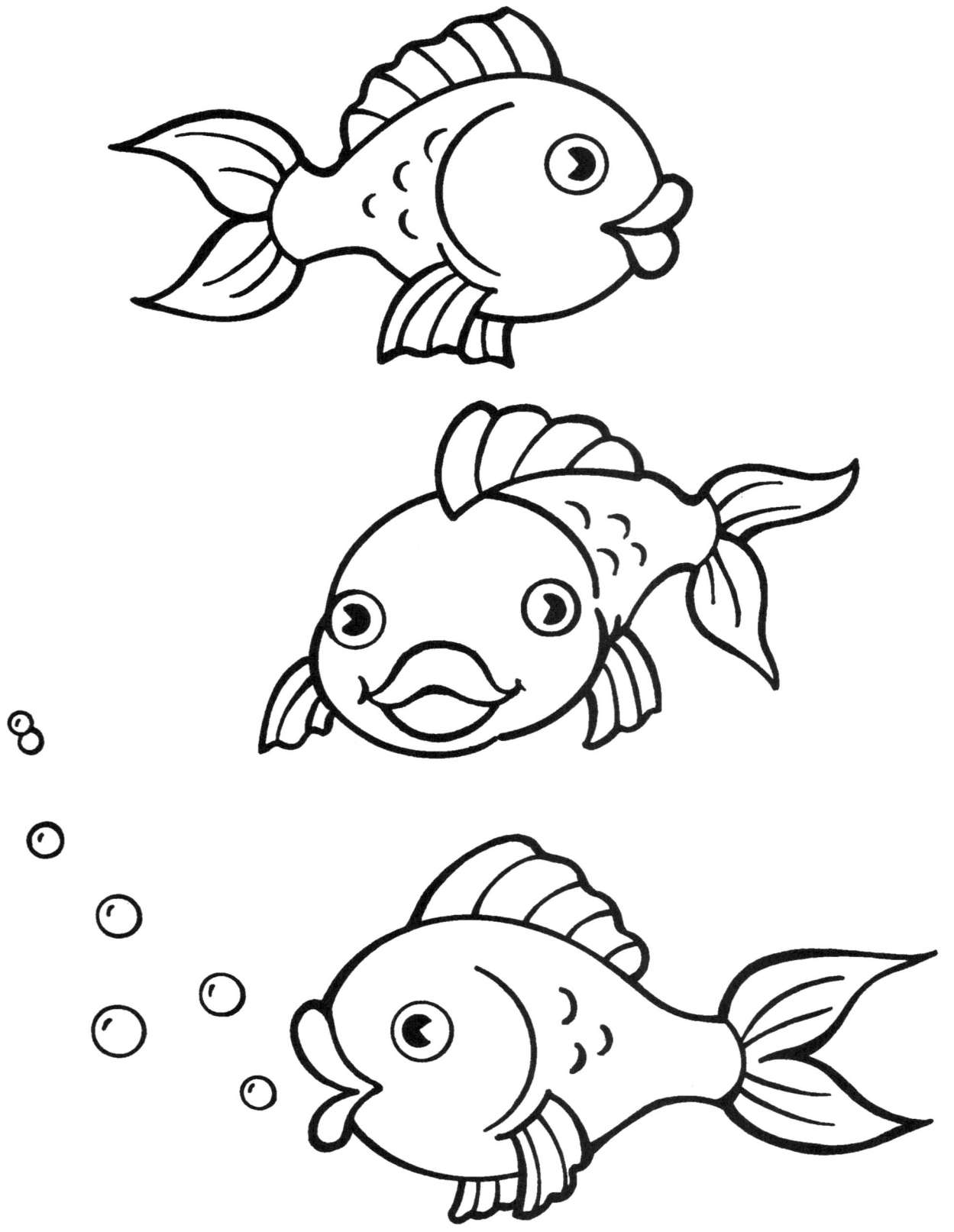

Fishy-Wishy

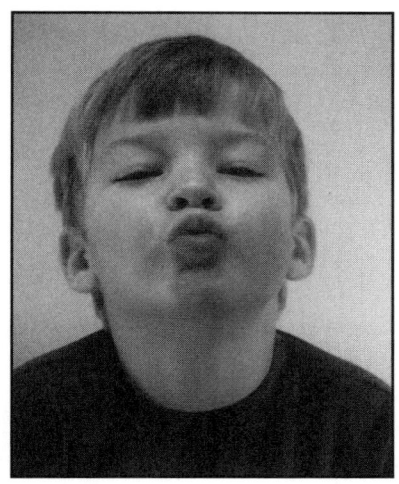

Fishy-wishy goes like this.

Make a series of exaggerated kisses.

Fishy-wishy gives a kiss.

Repeat the action.

Fishy-wishy blows a bubble.

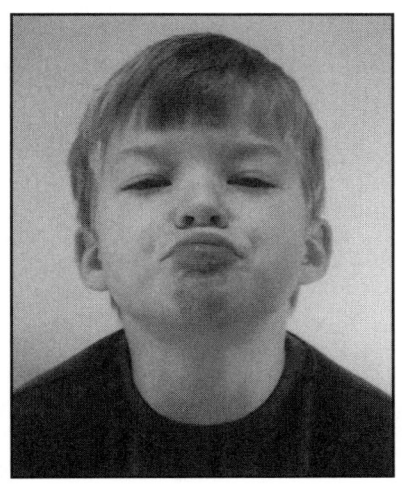

Purse lips and blow to make a "raspberry" noise.

Stop it, Fish! You'll get in trouble!

Dirt in Your Mouth

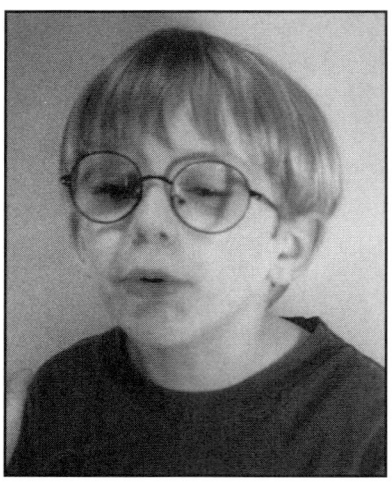

Don't put dirt in your mouth!
Spit it out!

Pretend to spit with a "pooh" motion.

Don't put bugs in your mouth!
Spit them out!

Repeat the action.

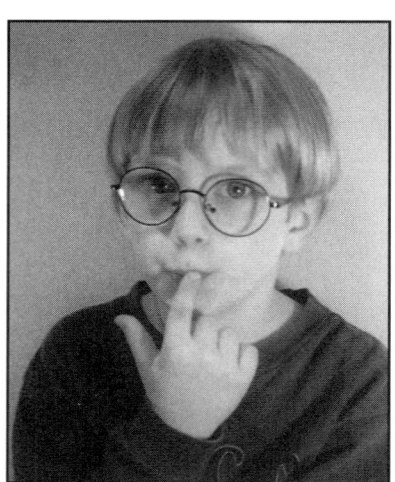

Don't put fingers in your mouth!
Spit them out!

Spit, spit, spit them,

Spit them out!

Touch each finger to mouth and "spit it away."

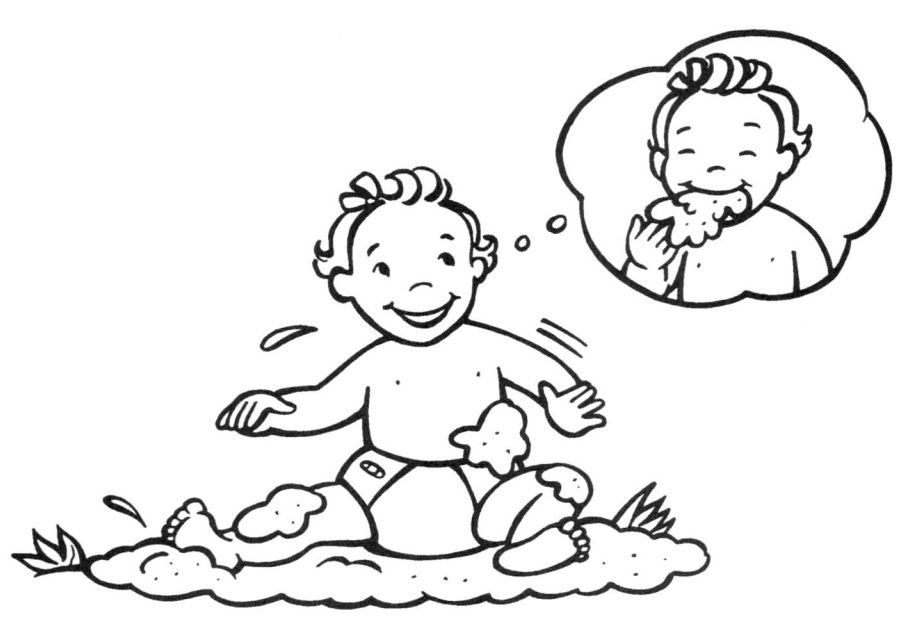

14

Flat Tire

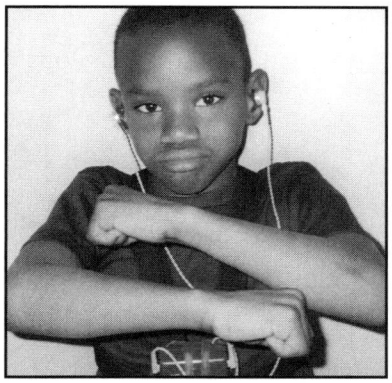

I'm a tire!

Here I go, down the road! Brrrrrrr!

Roll arms while making a soft "raspberry" noise.

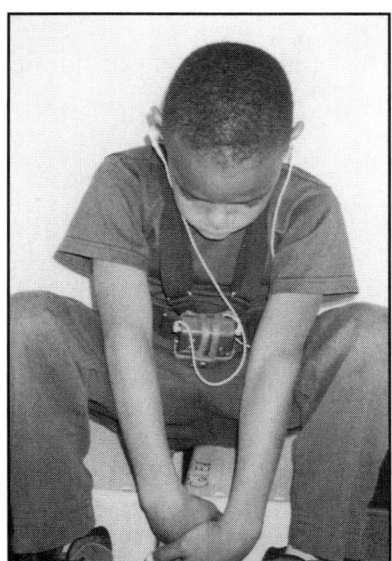

Uh-oh! I've got a flat!

Increase air pressure through lips to make a loud "raspberry" burst. Throw arms up in the air.

Resume rolling arms, but with a jerky motion. Make periodic raspberry bursts as the "flat tire" goes wobbly.

Drop arms to make continuous soft, expiring raspberry noises as head and arms go limp.

All flat! I'm stuck!

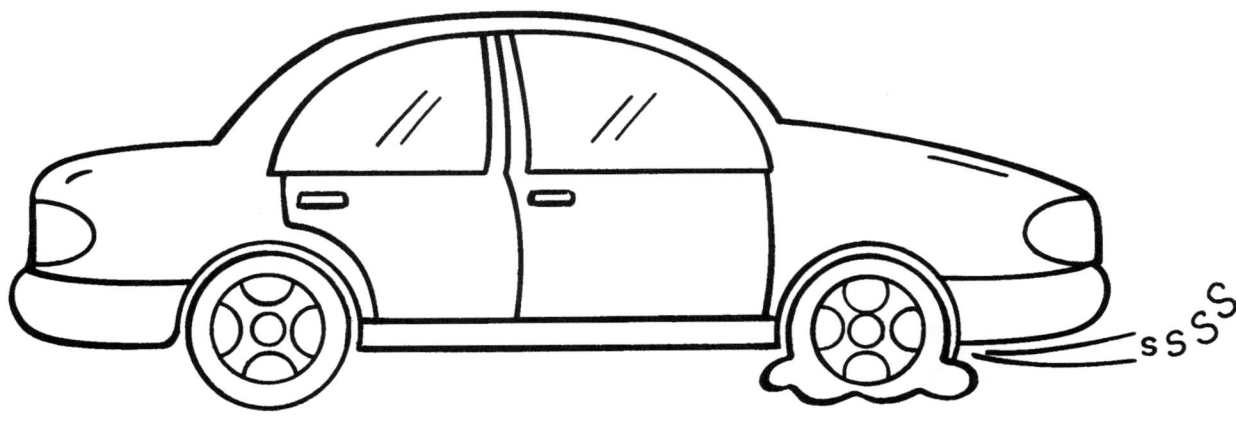

The Lost Mouth

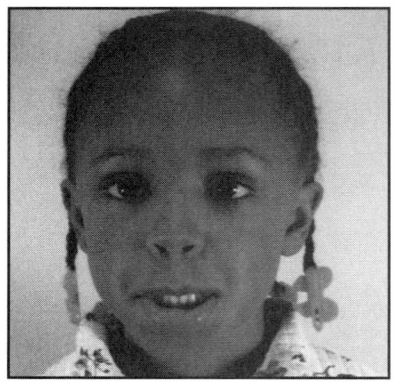

First, I lost my top lip. Oops!

Place bottom teeth over top lip.

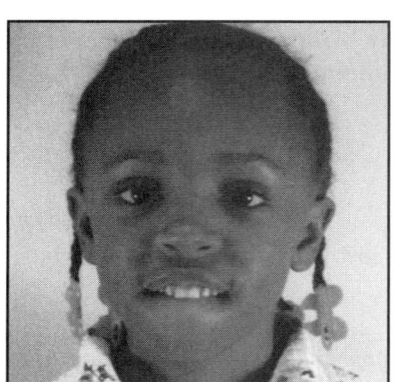

Then I lost my bottom lip. Eep!

Place top teeth over bottom lip.

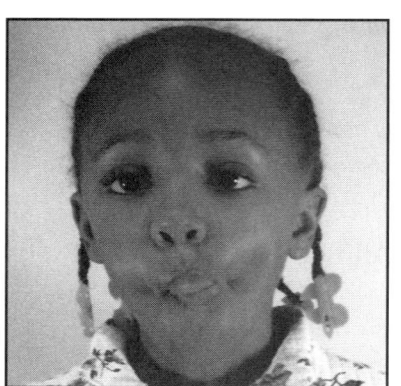

I looked, and both my cheeks were gone. Oh, my!

Suck in cheeks.

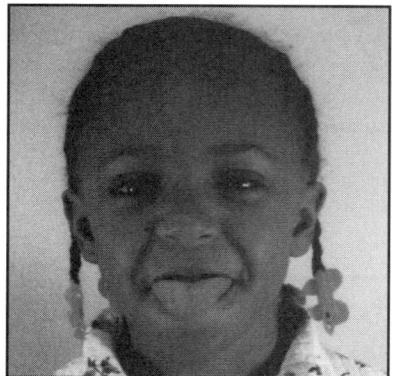

It got out! I lost my tongue!

Stick out tongue.

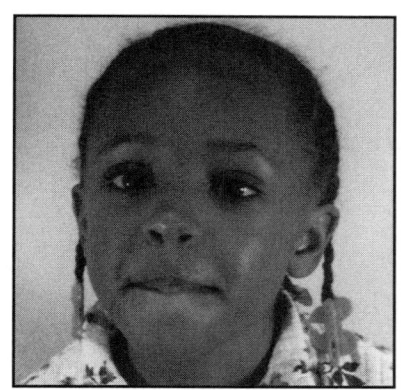

No more talking. Now I'm mum!

Suck in cheeks and lips and look sad.

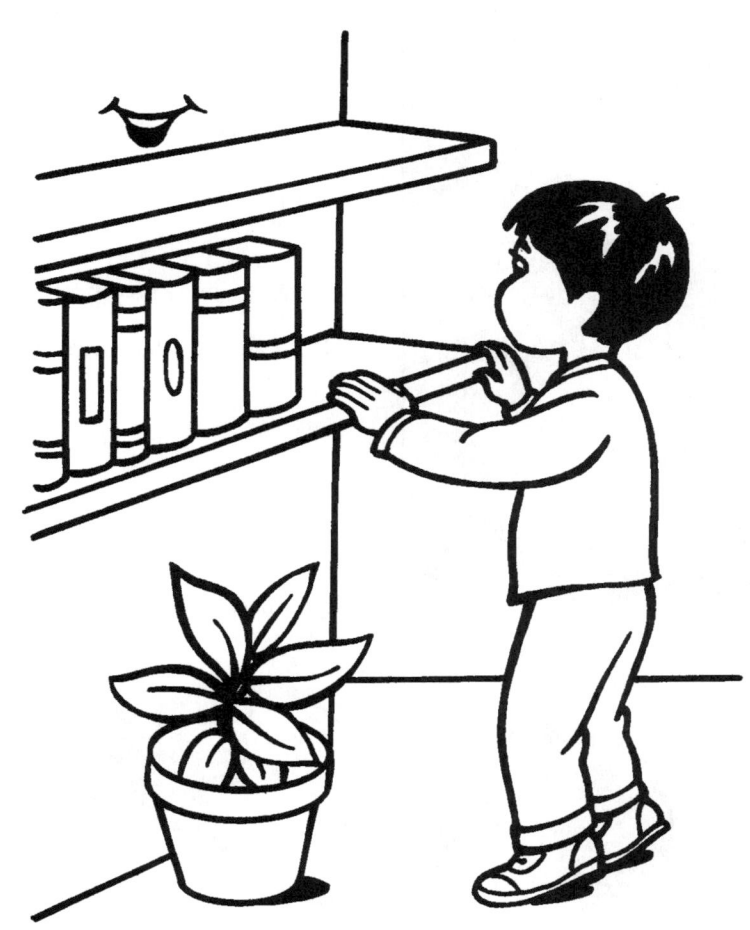

Kissy Missy, Kissy Mister

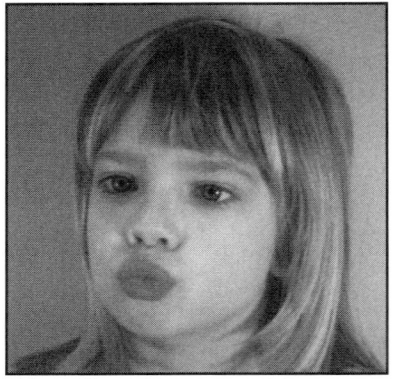

Kissy-kissy-kissy missy.

Pucker-kiss eight times.

Kissy-kissy-kissy mister.

Repeat the pucker-kiss eight times.

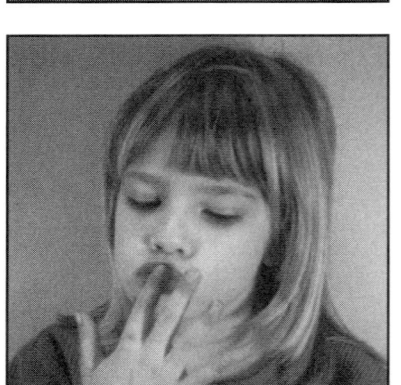

Kissy-kissy kissed her brother.

Hold up hands and pucker-kiss each fingertip for ten kisses.

Kissy-kissy kissed his sister.

Repeat the action, pucker-kissing each fingertip.

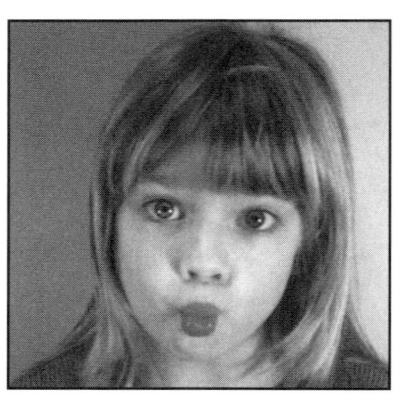

Kissy-kissy, kissy pout!
Turn those kisses inside out!

Suck in cheeks and protrude lips.

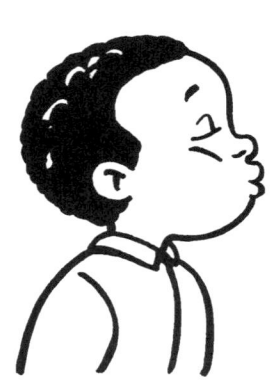
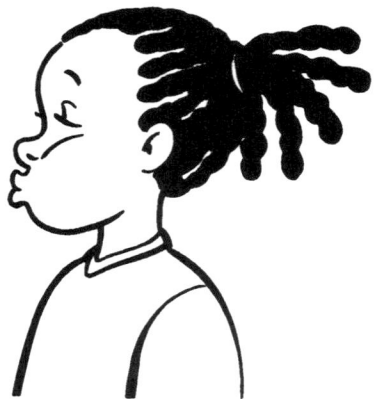

Peek-a-Boo Face

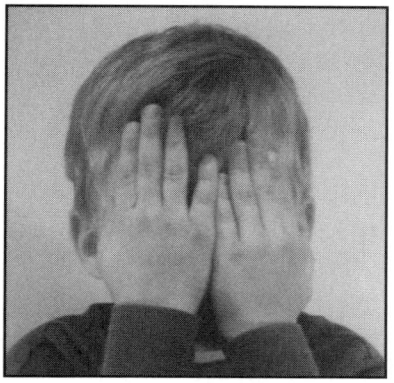

Cover and uncover your face while you tell this story. Then tell it again while the children cover and uncover their faces.

Close hands over face.

I had a toy.

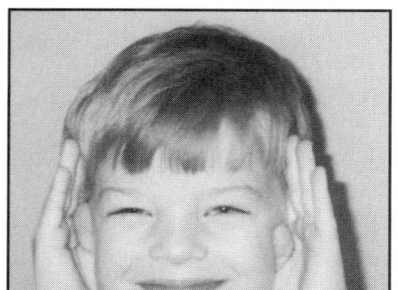

Open hands from face and show a smile. Close hands over face.

I lost it!

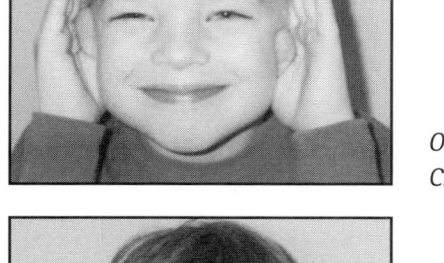

Open hands and show a frown. Close hands over face.

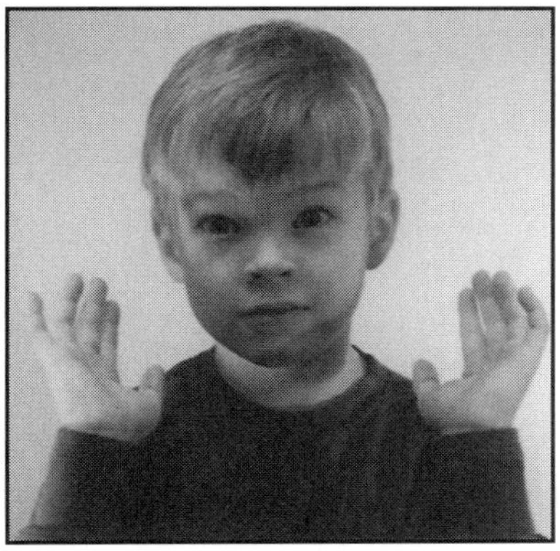

I looked for it. I found a monkey.

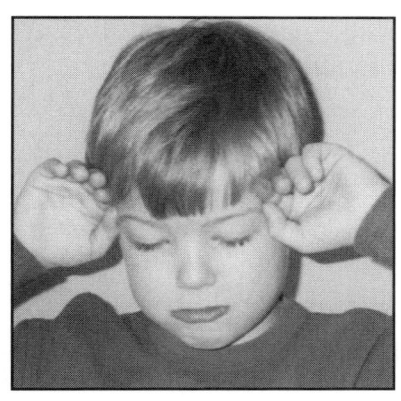

Open hands and show a surprised face. Close hands over face.

(continued)

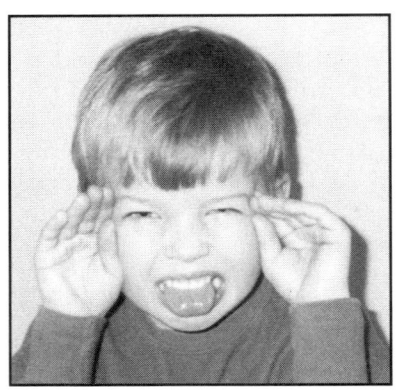

I found a bug.

*Open hands and show an icky face.
Close hands over face.*

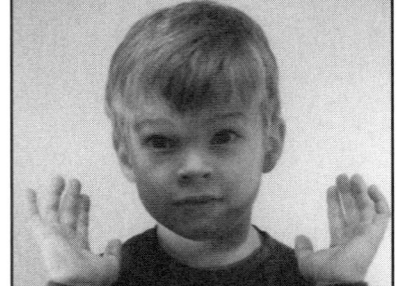

I found a button.

*Open hands and show a surprised face.
Close hands over face.*

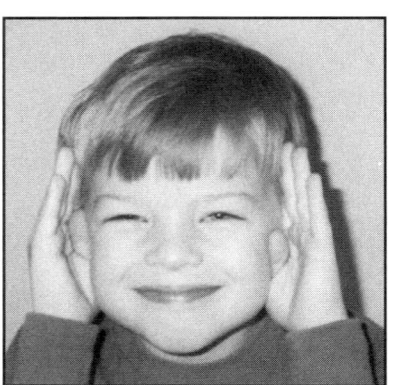

I found a friend.

*Open hands and show a smile.
Close hands over face.*

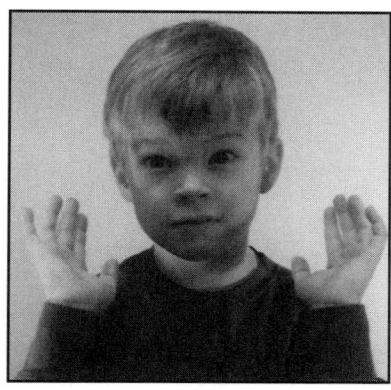

My friend found the toy!

Open hands and show a surprised face.

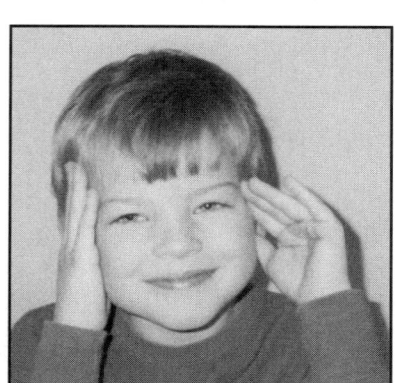

We played with it,
My friend and I.

Smile.

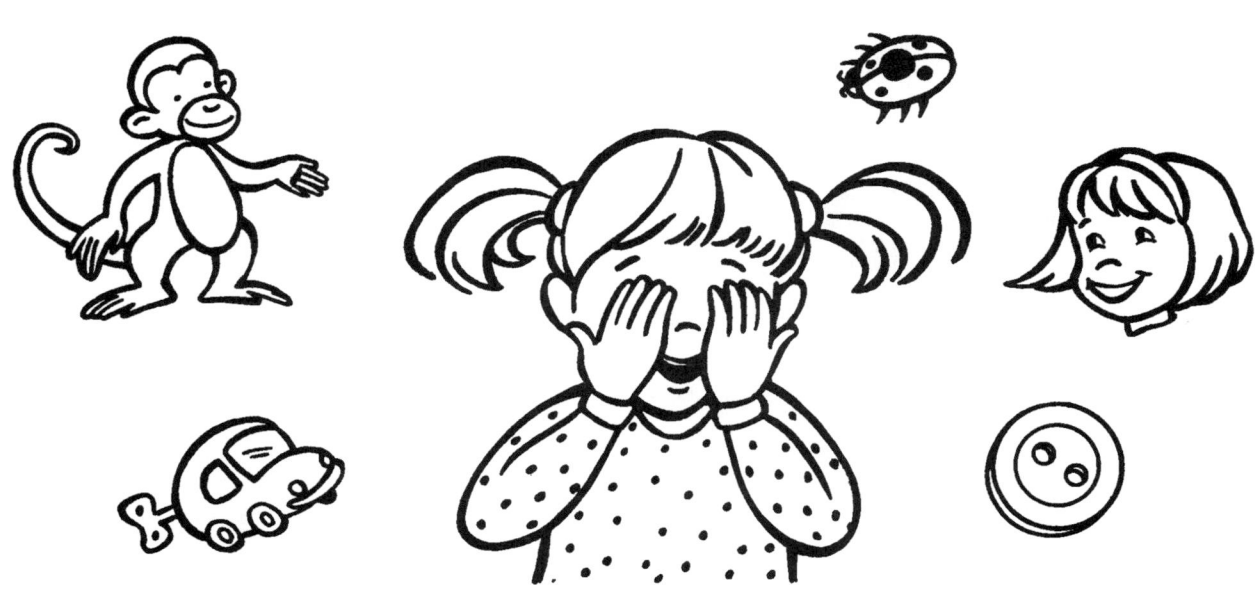

Driving the Car

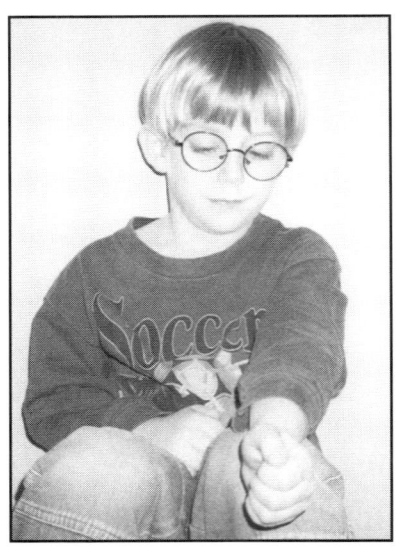

I am going to start the car.

Twist wrist, miming turning key in the ignition.

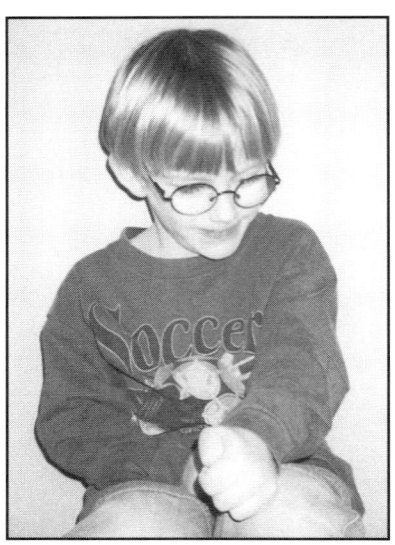

Rrrrrr!

Make an Rrrrr sound, then fade the noise into lip raspberries.

It didn't start.

Repeat the action and the sound, fading into lip raspberries.

It didn't start.

Repeat the action, but this time "rev up the engine." Make continuous loud raspberry sounds.

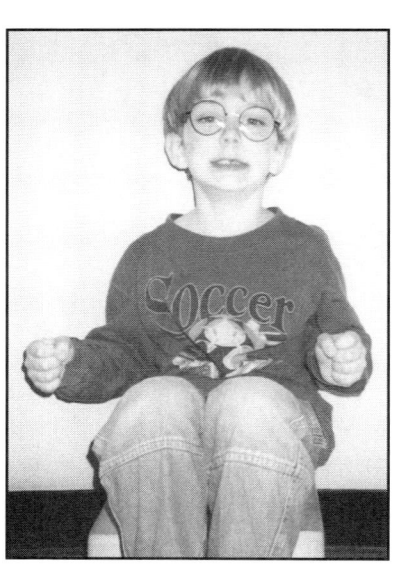

Reach forward and grasp an imaginary steering wheel. Pretend to drive.

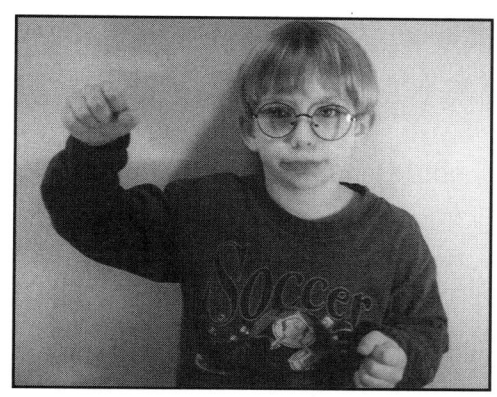

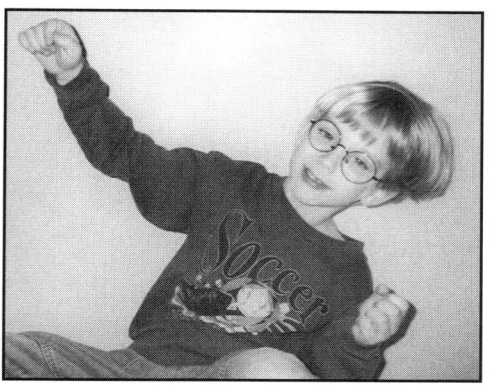

Take a hard left turn and lean far to the left. Continue to make raspberry sounds.

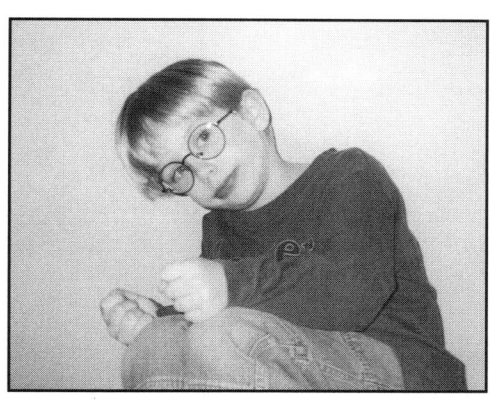

Repeat the action, turning to the right. Stretch the right foot forward and pretend to slam on the brakes. Make an exaggerated "Eeee" mouth shape as you grind to a halt.

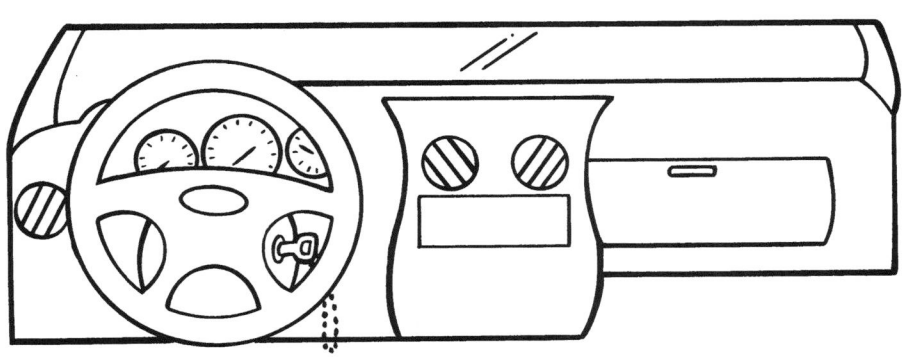

The Sneeze

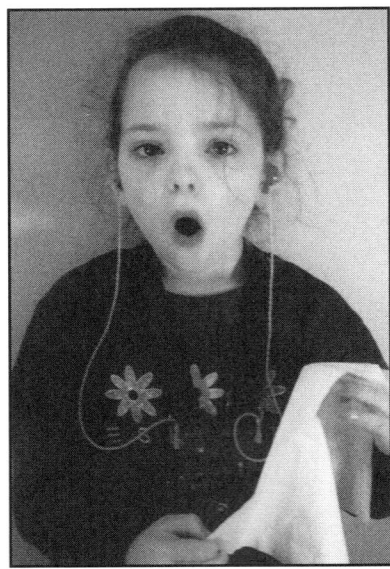

Give each child a face tissue.

Ooooo! Ooooo!

Form an exaggerated O with the mouth.

Eeeee! Eeeee!

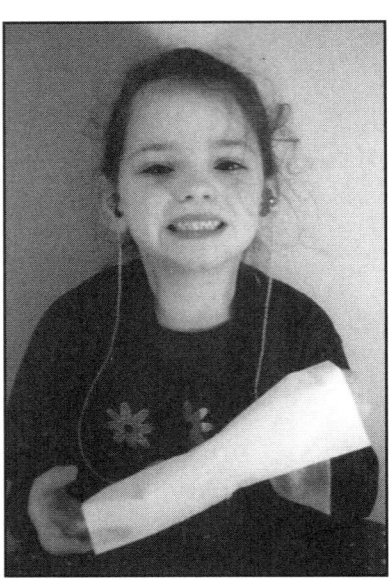

Form an exaggerated E with the mouth.

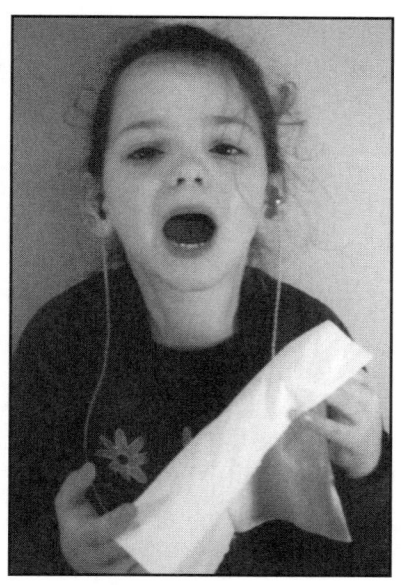

Ahhhh! Ahhhh!

Form an exaggerated AH with the mouth.

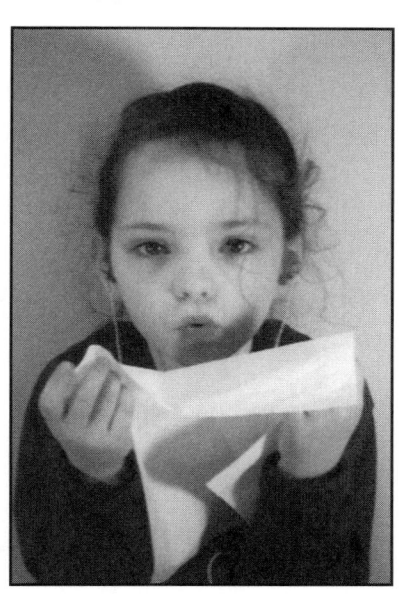

Choooo!

Blow into the tissue.

Excuse me!

Smiles and Frowns

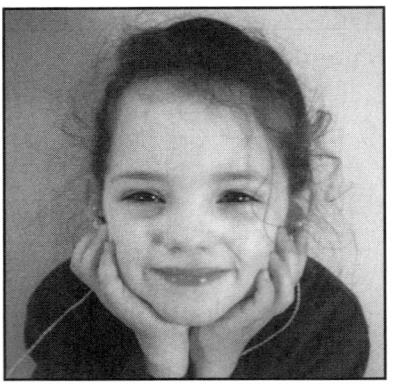

Smiles go up.

Show a big smile, keeping mouth closed.

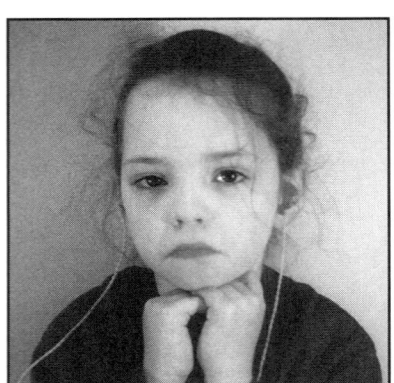

Frowns go down.

Show a big frown, with mouth turned down.

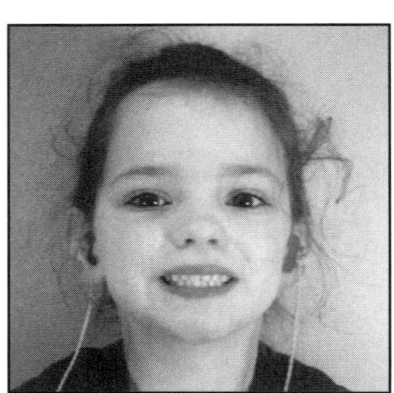

But grins go 'round and 'round and 'round!

Show a big, open-mouthed grin.

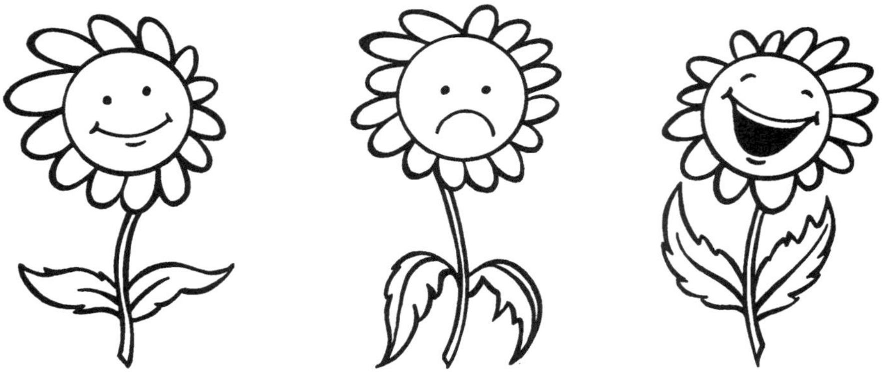

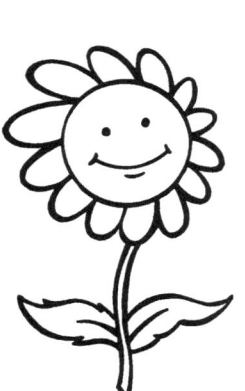  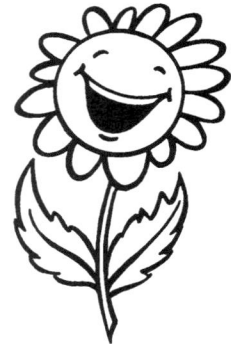

Cheeks

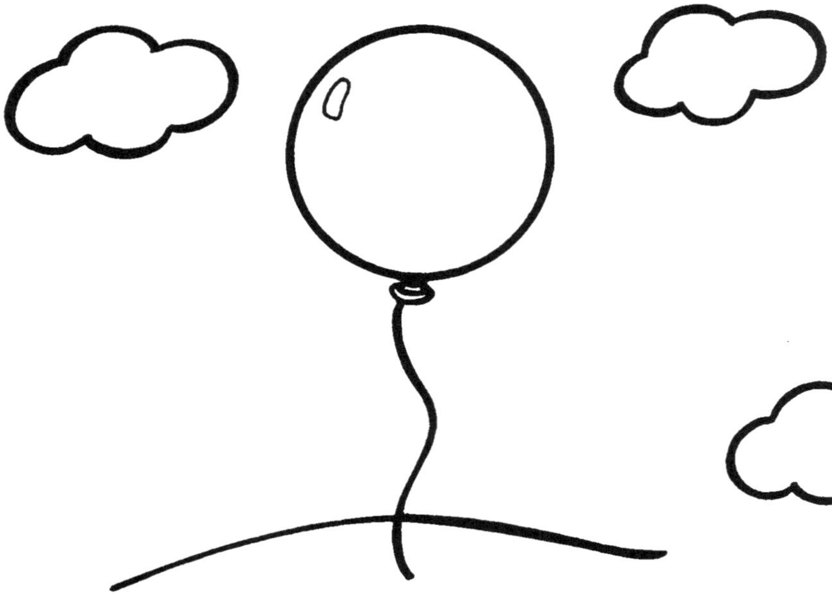

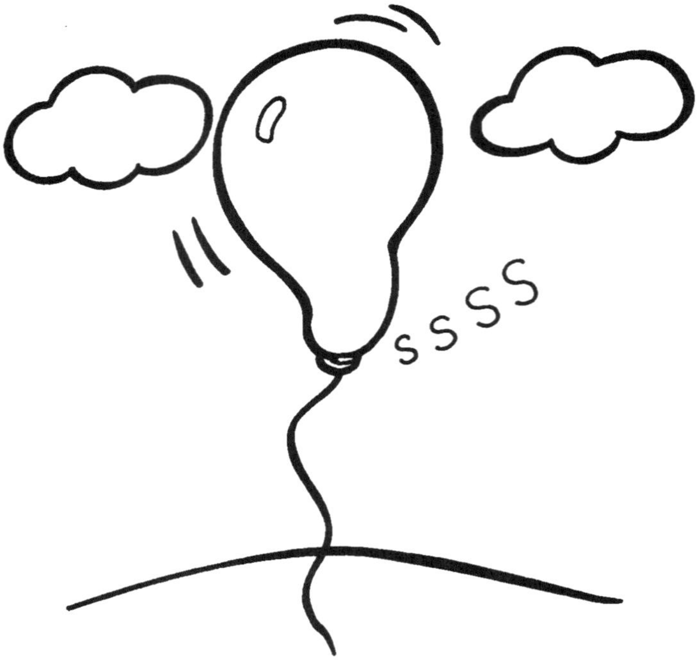

ssss

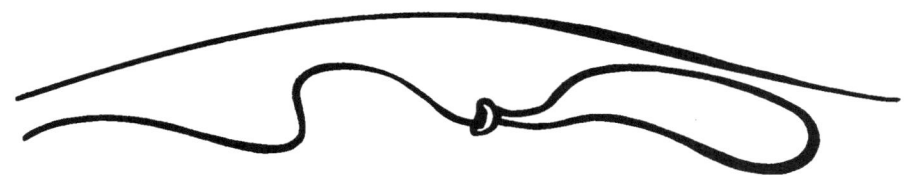

Balloon Blow

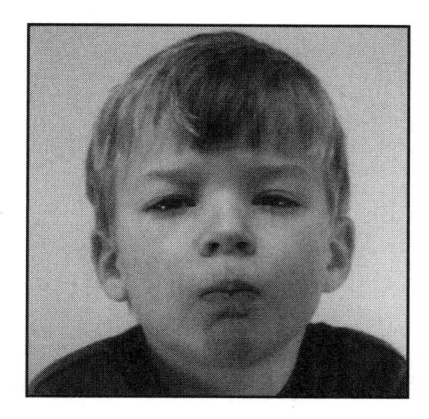

I am a balloon.

Take a deep breath and hold the mouth closed.

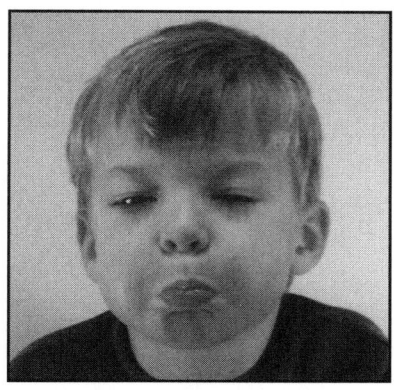

Take a deep breath and puff cheeks slightly.

Take a deep breath and puff cheeks larger.

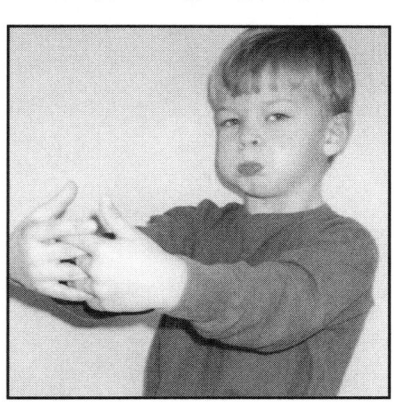

Take a deep breath and move to kneeling. Thrust chest forward, form a circle with the arms.

Take a deep breath and move to standing, chest thrust forward, cheeks puffed, eyes wide.

(continued)

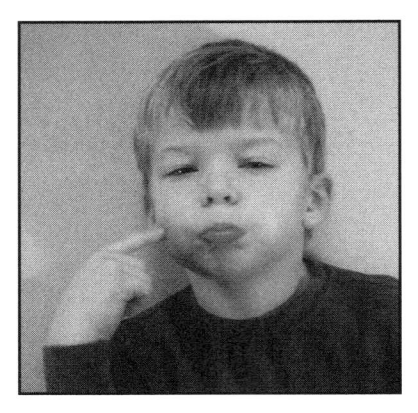

Press your finger to your cheek and release air.

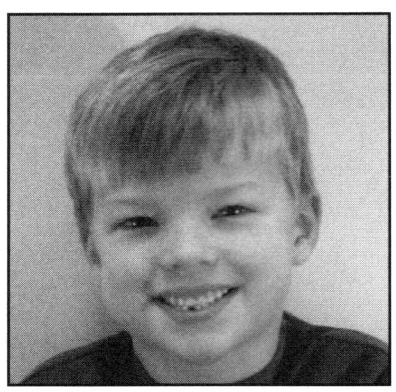

Position mouth and exaggerate lip retraction as you make an "sss" sound.

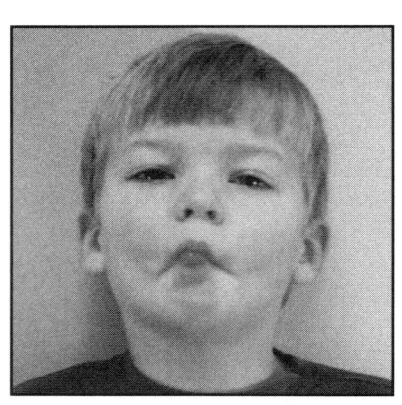

Sssssss.

Slowly return to floor.

Suck cheeks in.

All flat!

A Ball in Your Mouth

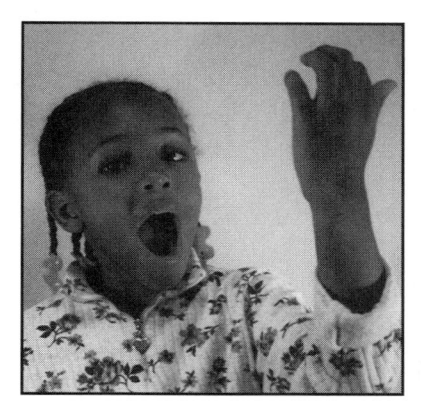

I have a ball. Watch me catch it.

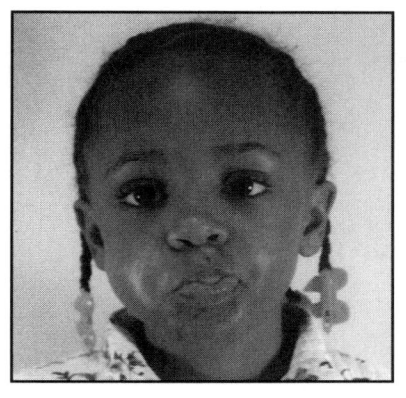

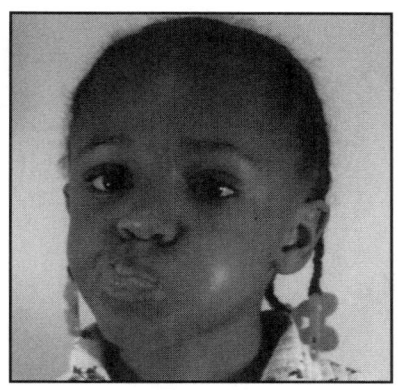

Mime an invisible ball. Pretend to throw it into the air and catch it in your mouth.

Fill your mouth with air and bulge one cheek, then the other, to mime the ball moving back and forth inside the mouth.

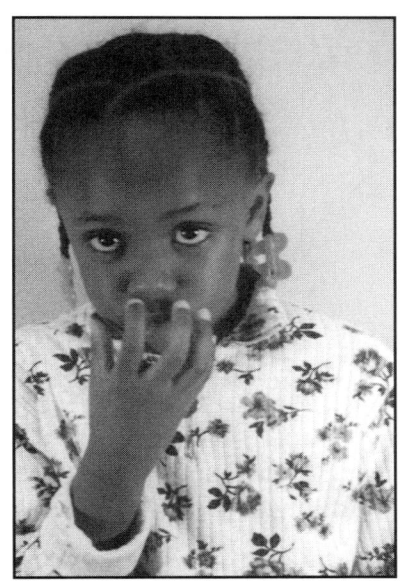

Open mouth and "puff" the ball into your hands.

Now it's your turn. Catch it with your mouth!

Pretend to toss the invisible ball to one of the children. The child pretends to catch it in the mouth and repeats the mime sequence.

Bubba's Bubble

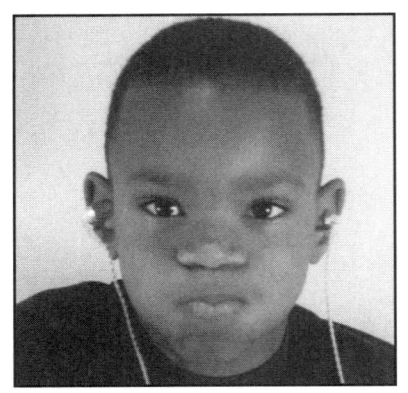

When Bubba blows a bubble,

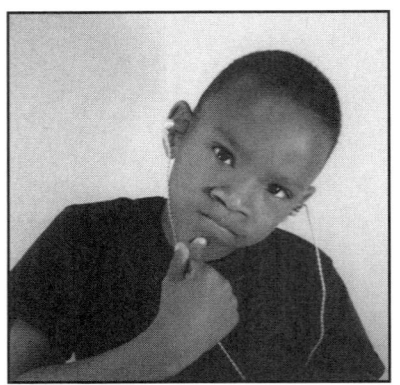

Blow up cheeks.

What happens next, please say.

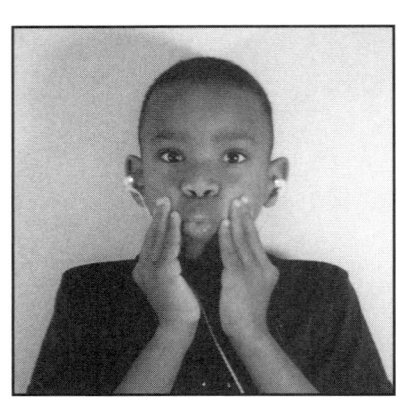

Put finger on chin.

Does Bubba's bubble burst?

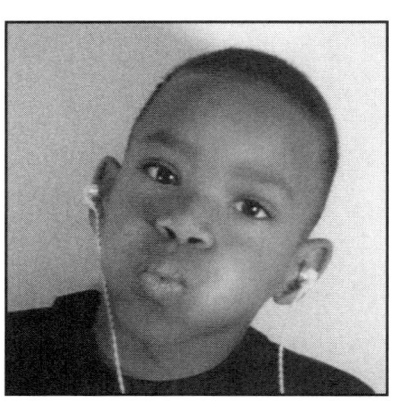

Clap cheeks.

Or does the bubble blow away?

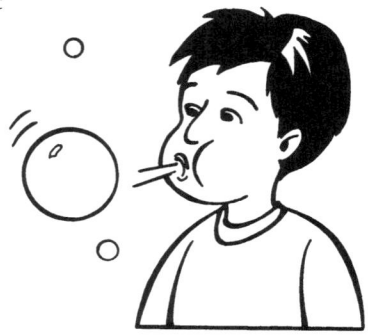

Blow.

Fat Cat

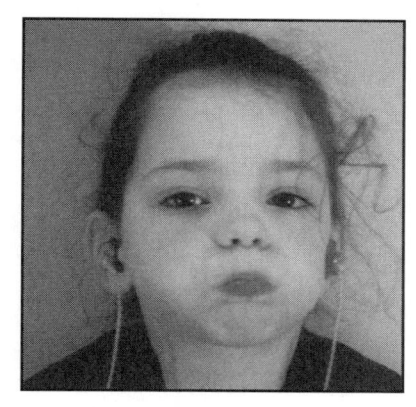

I met a cat.

Meow! Meow!

The cat was fat!

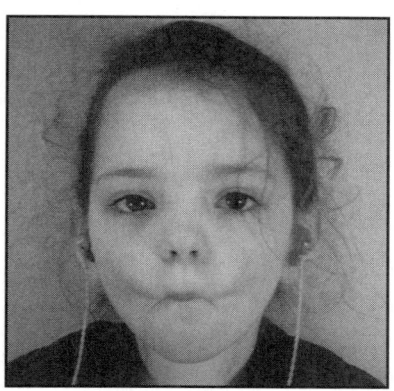

Puff out cheeks.

Meow!

A cat should not be fat like that!

Meow! Meow!

It should be slender, slim, and trim.

Suck in cheeks.

Meow!

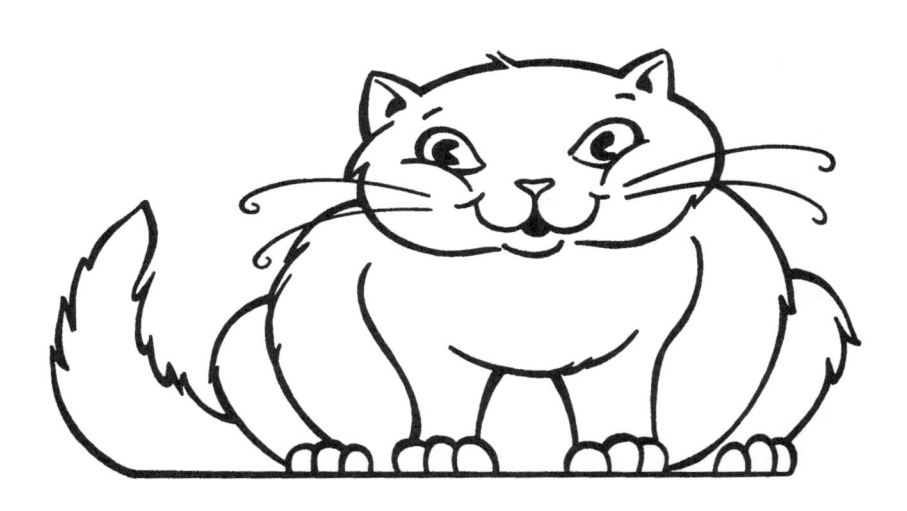

Dirty Eyeballs

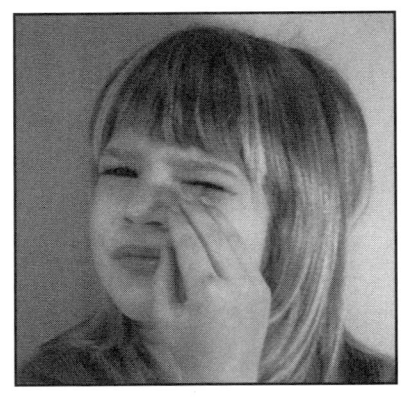

I have dirty, dirty eyeballs!

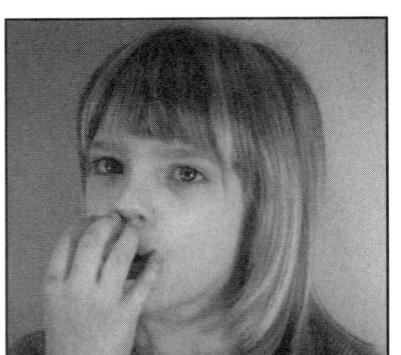

Close one eye and pretend to pop out an eyeball.

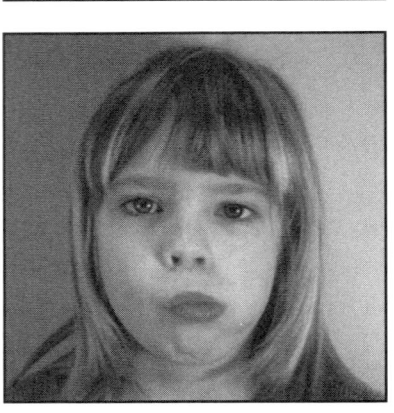

Pretend to put the eyeball in your mouth.

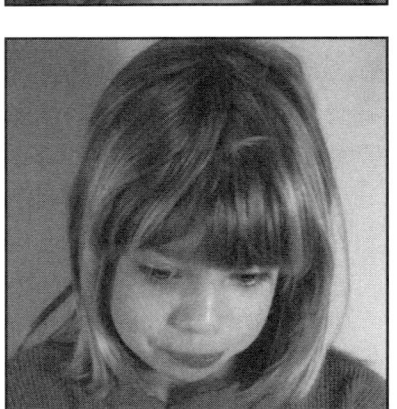

Run tongue inside the cheeks to create an illusion of something in the mouth.

Make an exaggerated swallow. Look surprised.

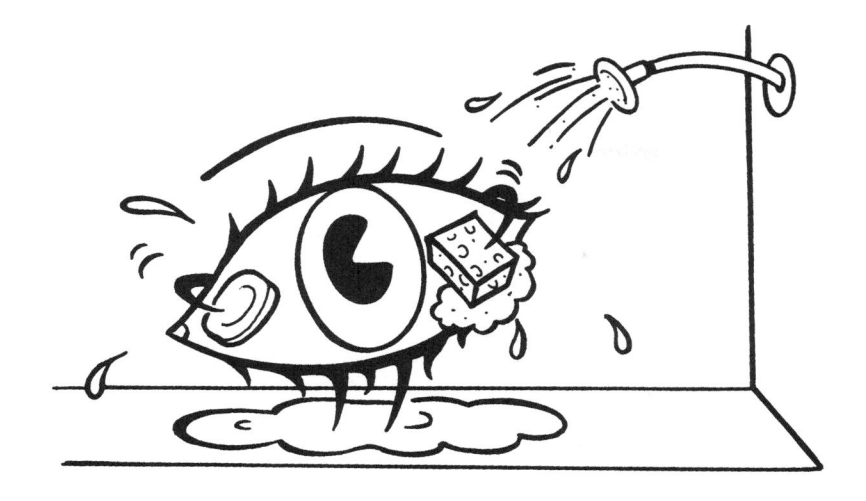

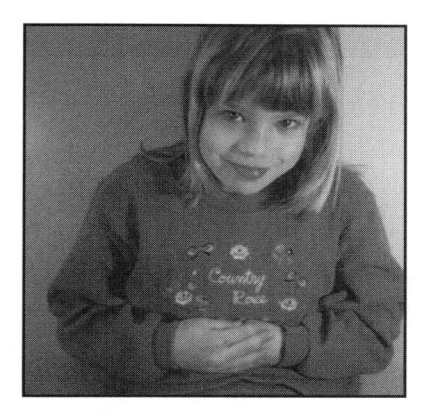

Push on your stomach with your hands. Eyes pop open.

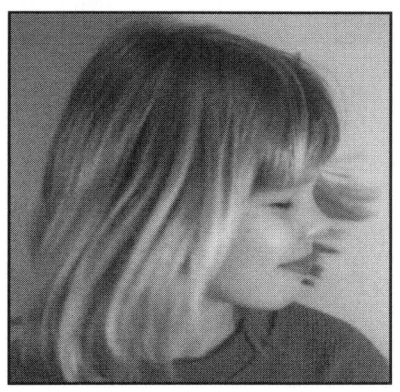

Shake head with eyes closed.

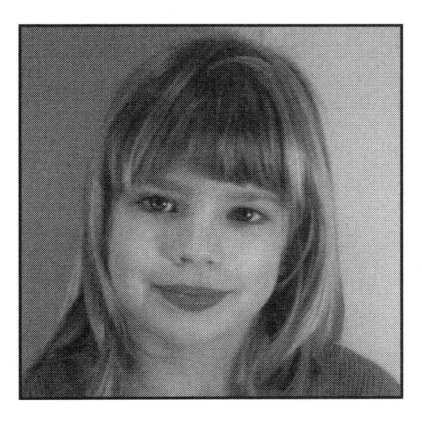

Open eyes.

Now they're OK!

The Fly

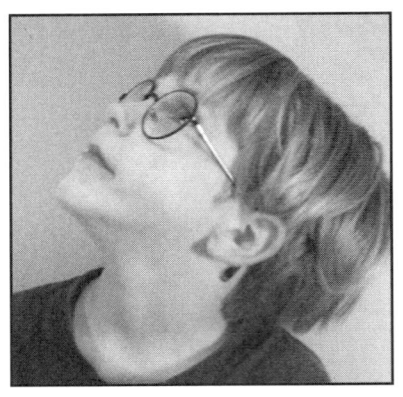

Zzzzzzzzzzzz!

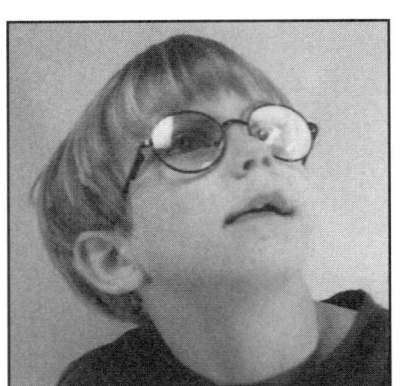

Turn head to watch fly.

There's a fly!

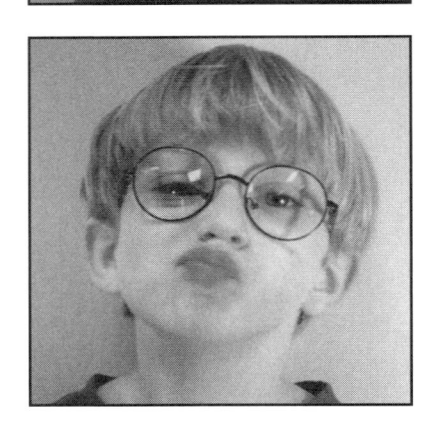

Continue to turn head, pretending to watch the fly.

I'll get it!

Bite the air and pretend to catch the fly in your mouth.

Mmmmmmmmm!

Pucker lips, make "mmmm" sound, and move lips in a circle as if the fly is moving around inside the mouth.

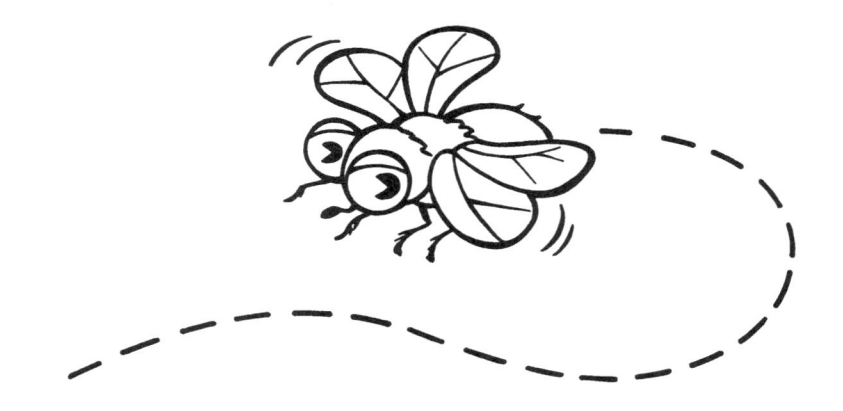

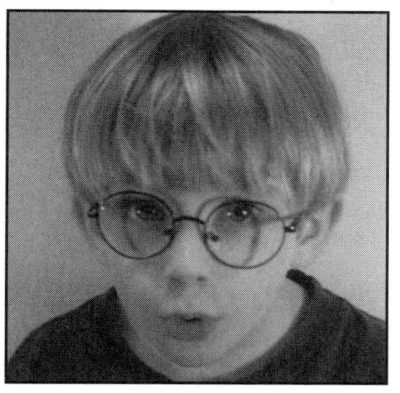

Pi-tooey!

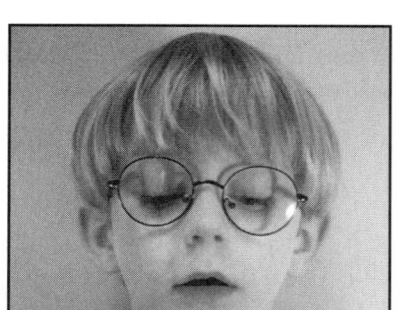

Pretend to spit out the fly.

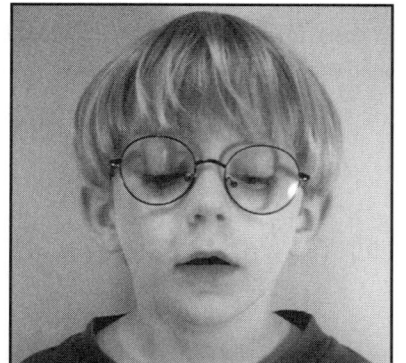

Zzzzzzzzzzzzzz!

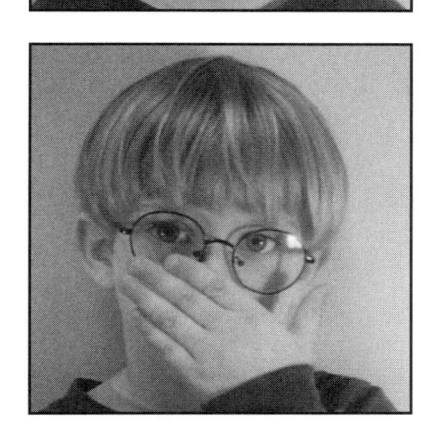

Pretend to watch the fly again. Pretend the fly lands on your nose. Look at the end of your nose.

I'll get it!

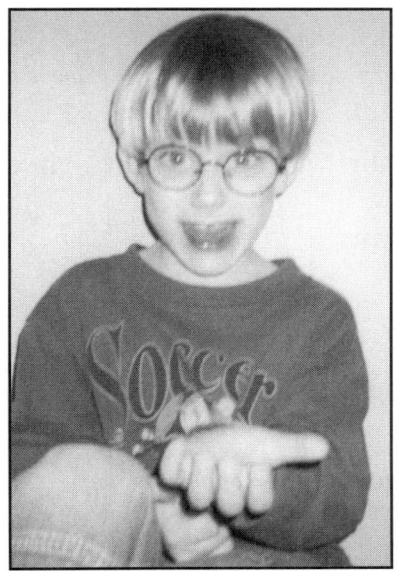

Take careful aim and bring your hand to your nose.

Yuk!

Pull hand from face, look at palm as if the fly is there, and make exaggerated "yuk" expression.

The Worm

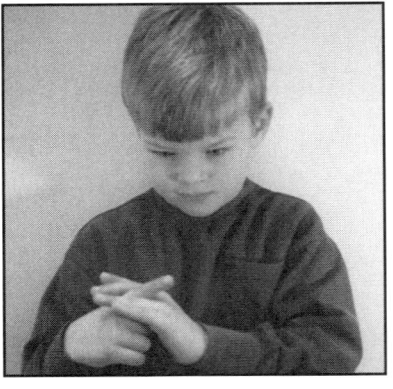

One day, a little worm crawled up from its home in the ground. It poked its head out three times.

Poke your index finger through the fingers of your other hand to mime the worm. Let the worm poke its head out three times. Count.

1. . . 2. . . 3.

I ate the worm!

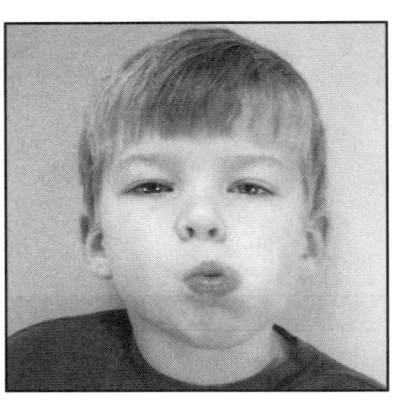

Pretend to eat the worm.

Help! It's trying to get out! Watch it poke my left cheek.

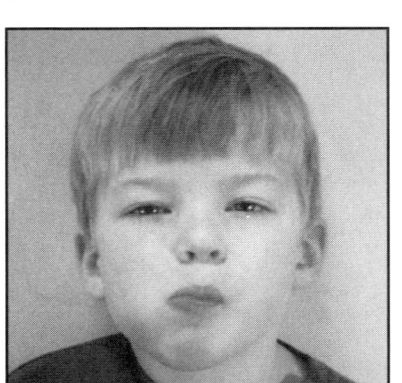

From inside the mouth, poke tongue in left cheek.

Now watch it poke my right cheek.

From inside the mouth, poke tongue in right cheek.

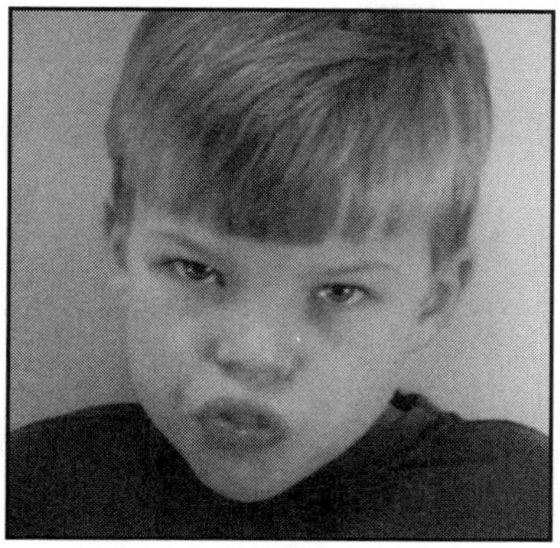

Watch the worm go around and around.

From inside the mouth, run tongue in a circle behind lips.

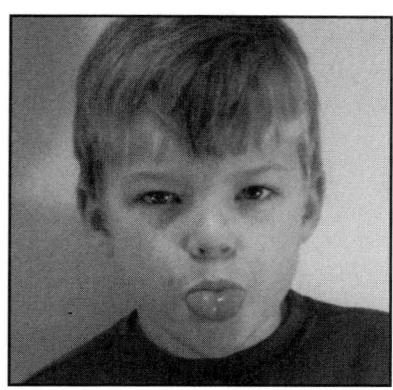

Ooops! It got away!

Stick out tongue.

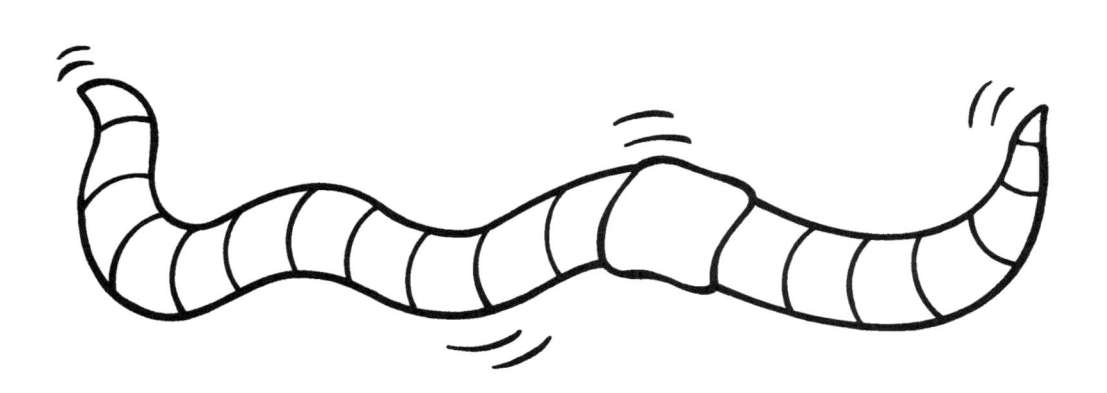

Toadie Fingers

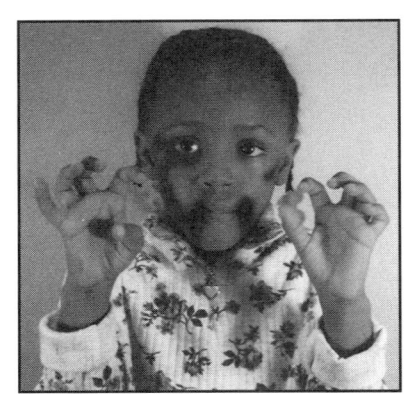

Never ever touch a toad!
Touch a toad, and I am told
You'll grow a hairy, scary wart!
Toadie fingers, toadie fingers
Grow a hairy, scary wart!

Hold hands up in front of face and wiggle fingers.

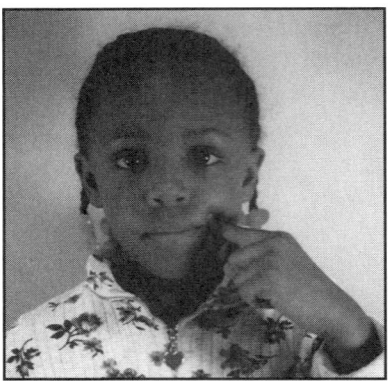

Touch index finger to right cheek.

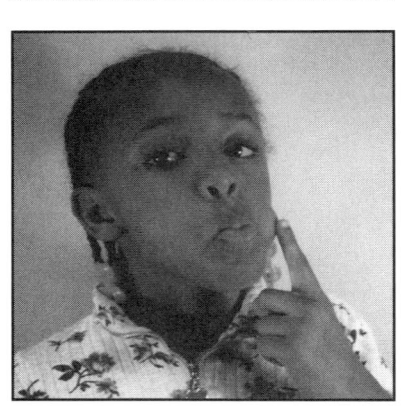

From inside your mouth, push your tongue on your cheek under your finger, making a bump (a "wart") in your cheek. Scream in horror. Repeat with warts in different spots.

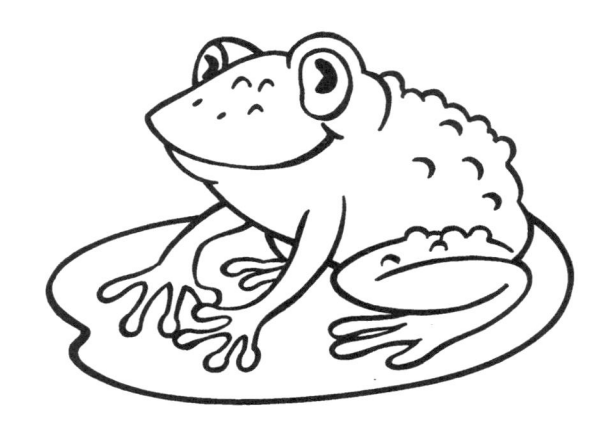

Tongue

The Butterflies

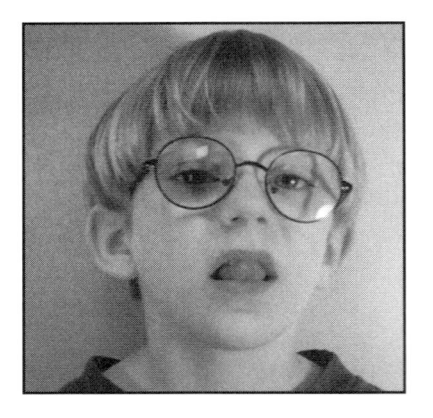

The butterflies will flutter by
And move their little tongues.
They flick, they lick.

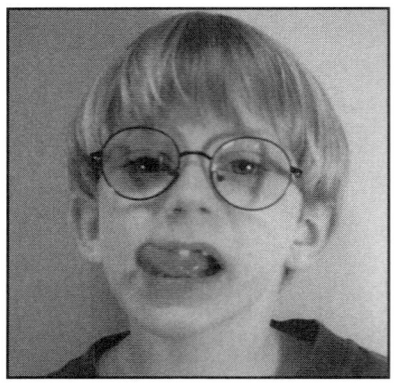

Flutter tongue in and out of mouth.

They move them all around.

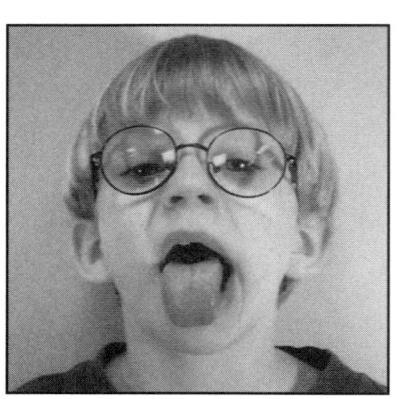

Move tongue in circle around open lips.

They touch them to the flowers
And drink without a sound.

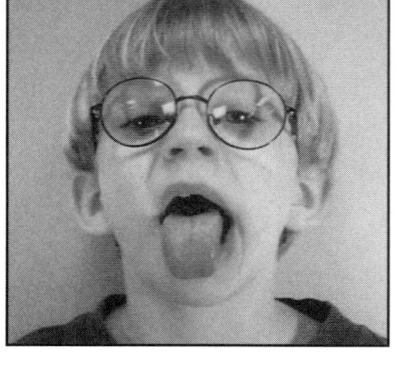

Flutter tongue in and out of mouth.

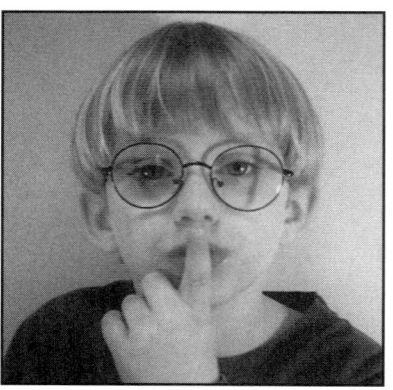

Shhh!

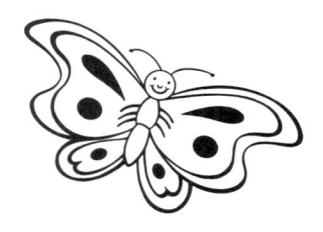

Place your finger to your lips as you say, "Shhh!"

Button Head

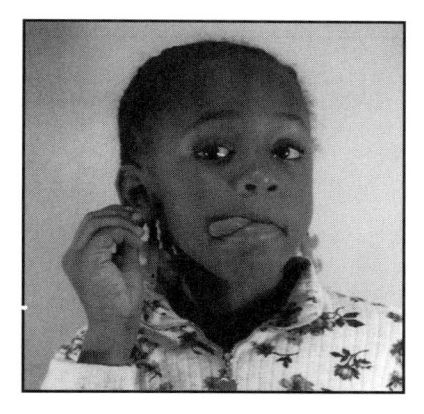

I have a button head,
A button head, a button head.
I have a button head.
Watch me push my buttons.

Tug right ear; protrude tongue slightly from right side of mouth.

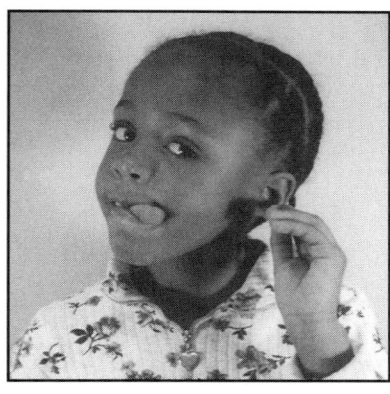

Tug left ear; protrude tongue slightly from left side of mouth.

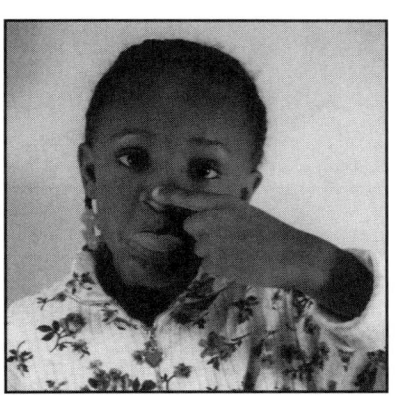

Push nose; protrude tongue from the center of mouth.

Repeat the actions, varying the sequence as interest permits.

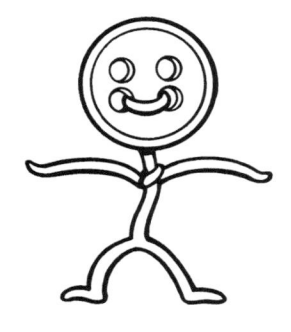

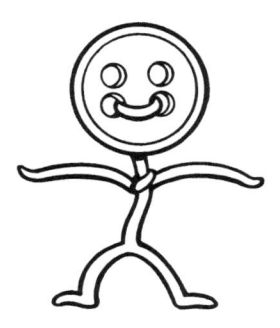

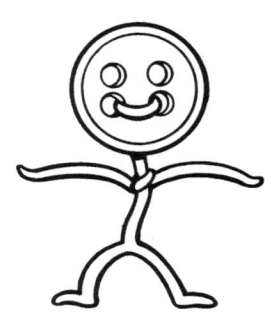

Careful Willie

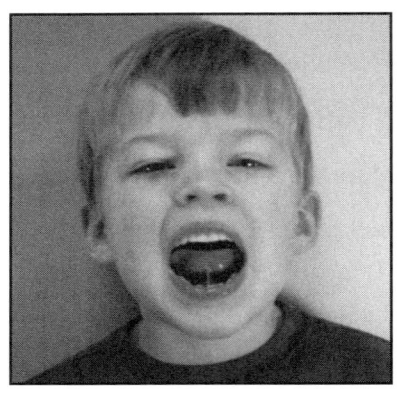

Careful Willie is a mole.

Careful Willie lives in a hole.

Open mouth slowly and dramatically. Elevate and wiggle tongue inside mouth.

Willie's hole has monstrous teeth,

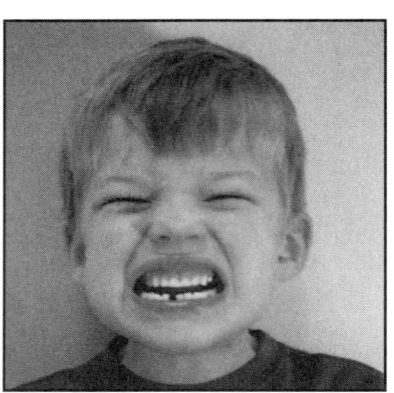

Bare teeth.

Sharp on top,

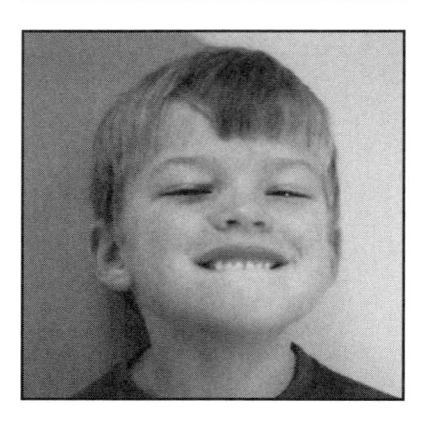

Place top teeth over bottom lip,

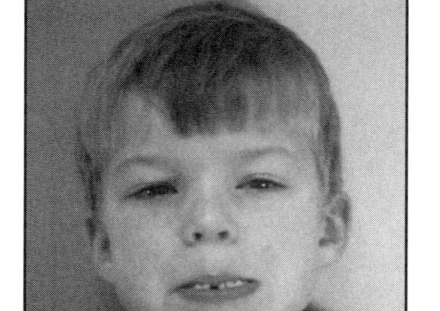

And sharp beneath.

then bottom teeth over top lip.

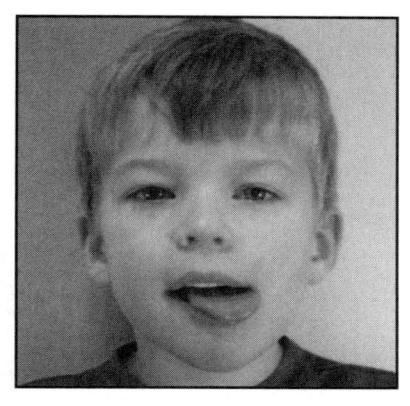

Careful Willie wants to play.
Willie wants to see the day.
Quietly creeping, he comes out.
Careful Willie looks about.
He looks left.

Protrude tongue to the left side of mouth.

He looks right.

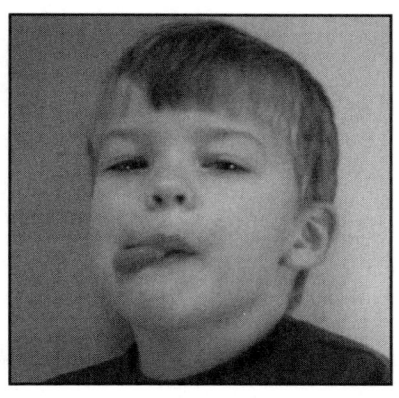

Protrude tongue to the right side of mouth.

He looks left. He looks right.

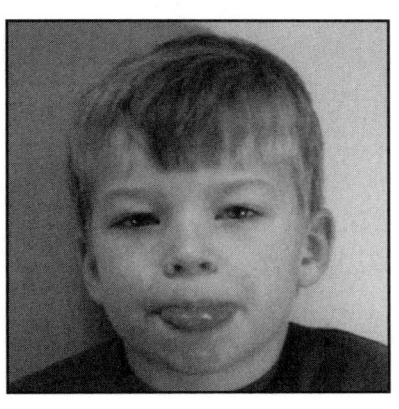

Move tongue from left to right side of mouth several times.

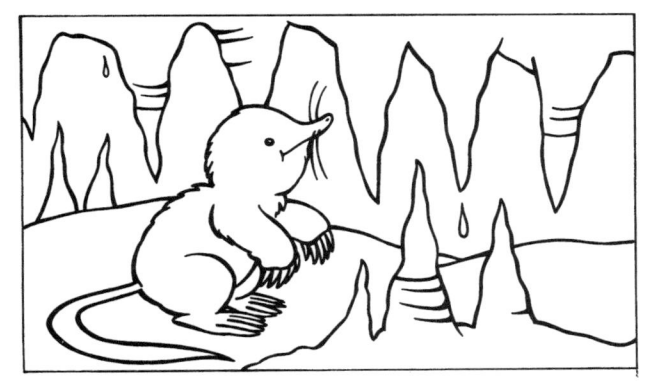

He looks left. He looks right.

Repeat the action.

I think I'll keep him in tonight.

Close mouth on Willie.

I Can Count My Teeth

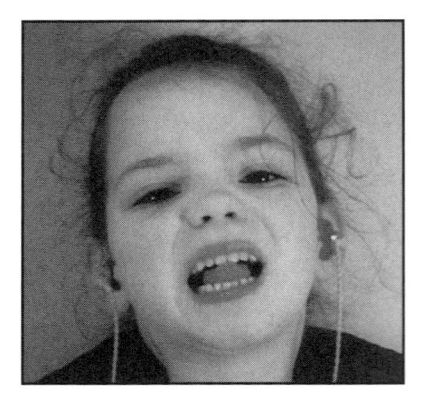

I can count my teeth.

1. . . 2.

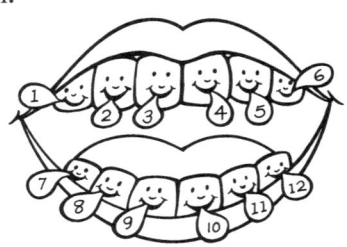

Place tip of tongue on incisors, one by one.

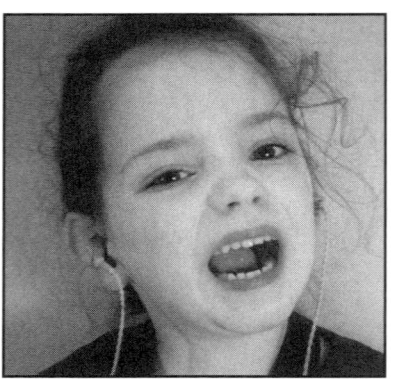

I can count my teeth.

Can you?

Place tip of tongue on other teeth, one by one.

I can count them with my tongue.

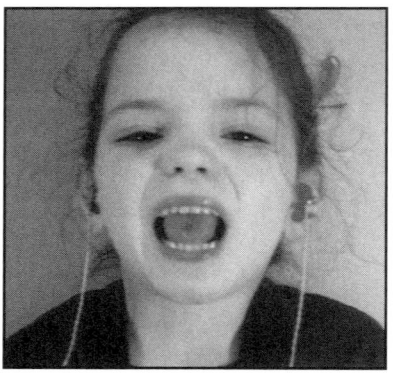

Continue to "count" teeth.

But I can't bite until I'm done!

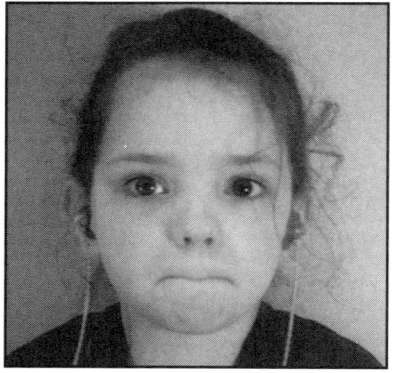

Pull tongue into mouth and close lips.

Whew!

The Super-Clean Worm

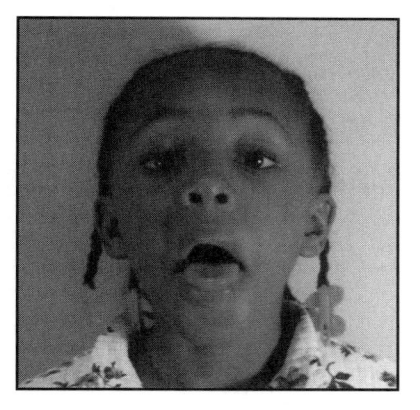

There once was a super-clean worm

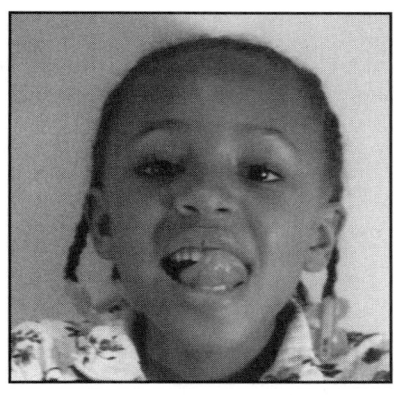

Open mouth and protrude tongue.

Who hated the thought of a germ.
She cleaned all her teeth
On top and beneath

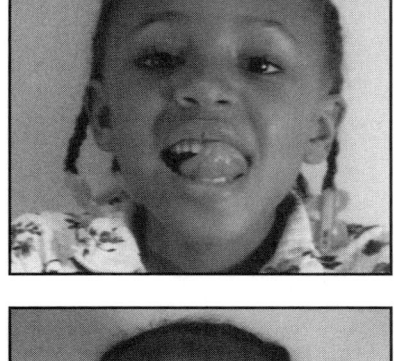

Run tongue back and forth over top teeth, then bottom teeth.

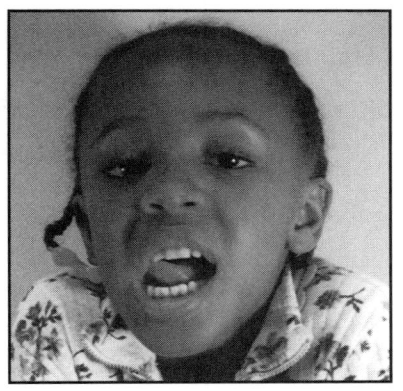

And everywhere else she could squirm.

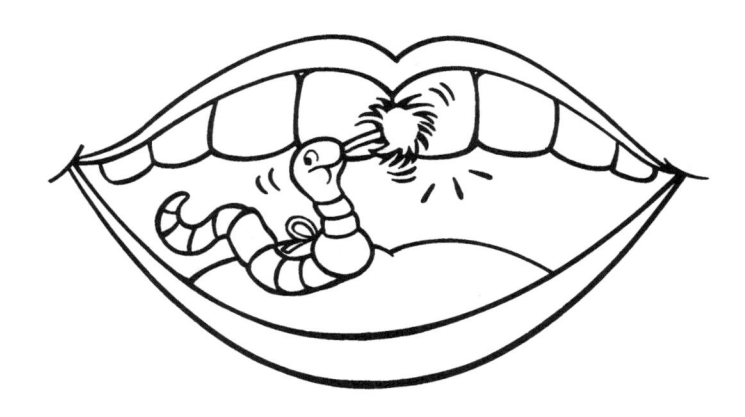

Twist tongue back into the mouth and run it over back teeth.

Momma Kitty

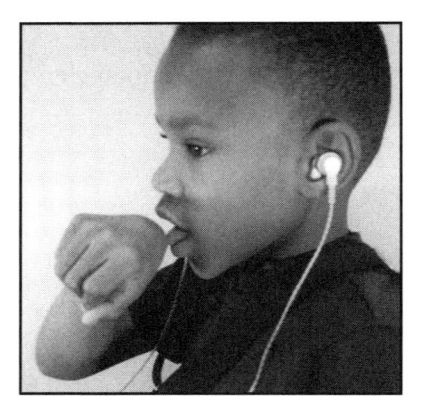

Momma Kitty cleans her kits
With tiny little kitty licks.
She licks, licks, licks their little paws.

Pretend to lick back of hands.

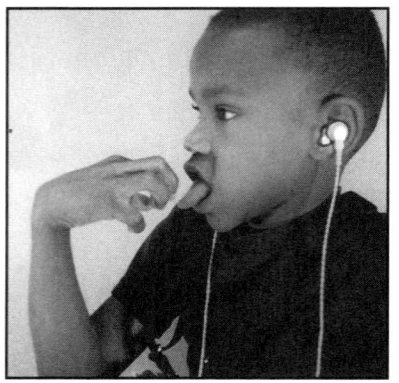

She washes out their tiny claws.

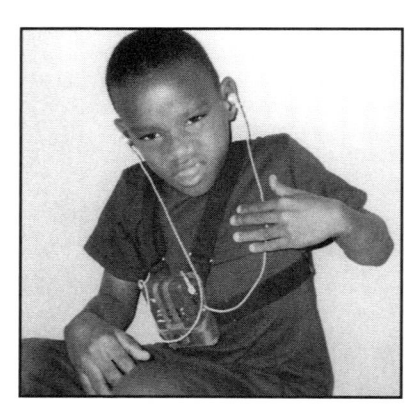

Curl fingers into claws and pretend to lick them.

I am glad I'm not a kitty.
Kitty washing makes me sticky!

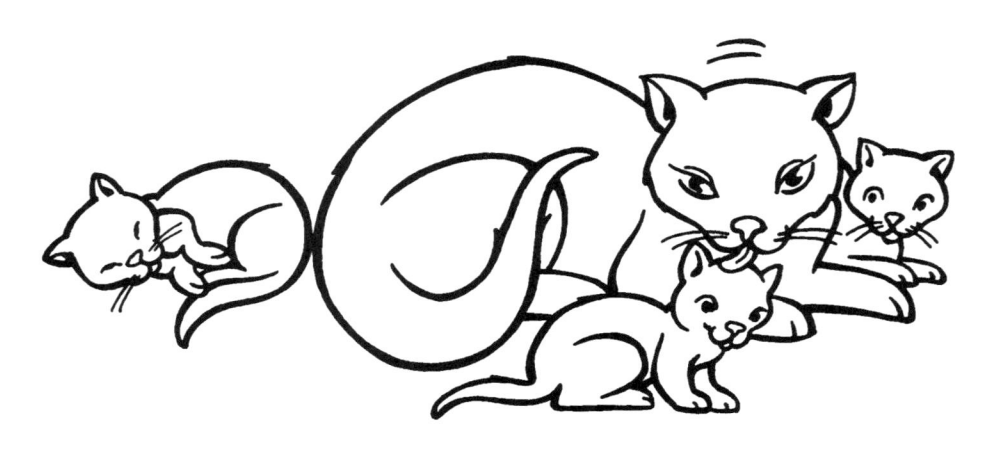

Make a "yuk" face and wipe hands on thighs.

About Snakes

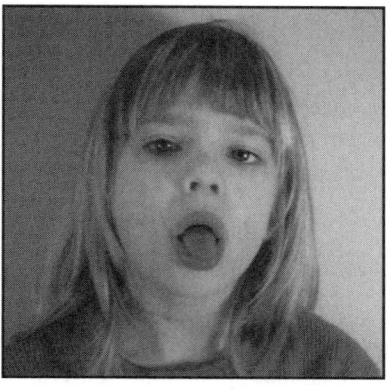

A snake smells with its tongue.

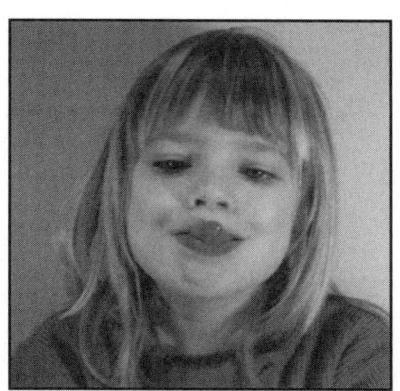

Protrude tongue and make it flicker.

A snake smells with its tongue.

Repeat the action.

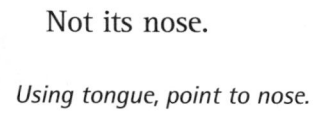

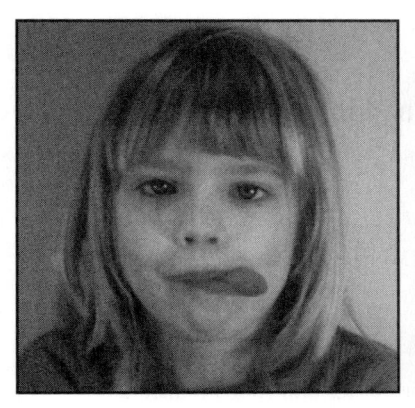

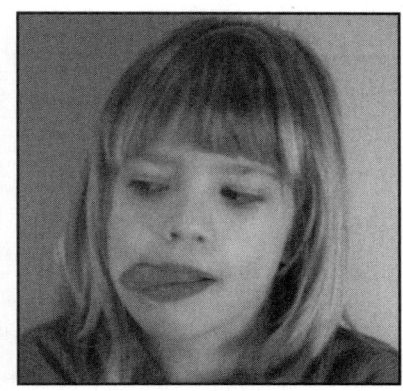

Not its nose.

Using tongue, point to nose.

Not its ears.

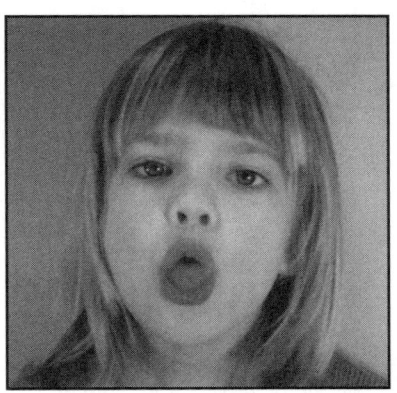

Using tongue, point to each ear.

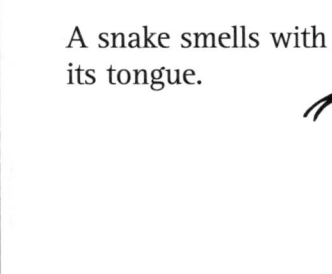

A snake smells with its tongue.

Flicker tongue and shudder.

This Little Piggy
Traditional Nursery Rhyme

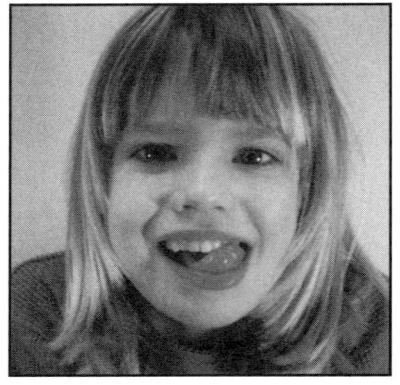

This little piggy went to market.

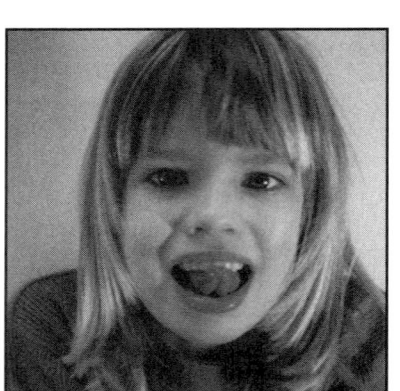

Open mouth and touch a tooth on the left side of your mouth with your tongue.

This little piggy stayed home.

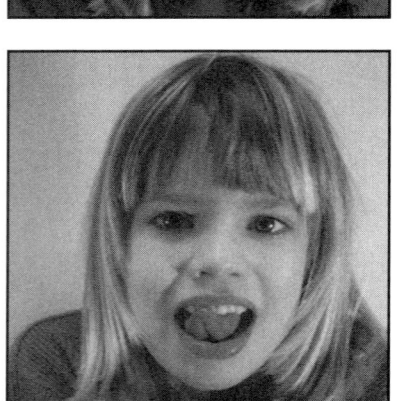

Move your tongue to the right and touch a different tooth with your tongue.

This little piggy had roast beef.

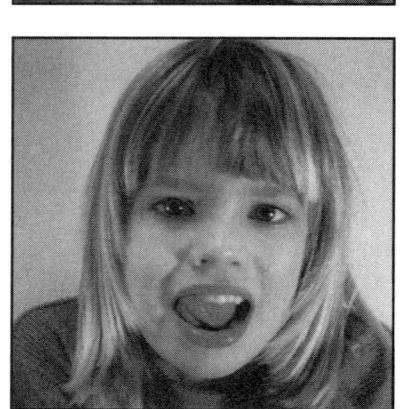

Move your tongue to the center and touch a different tooth with your tongue.

This little piggy had none.

Continue moving your tongue to the right and touch a different tooth with your tongue.

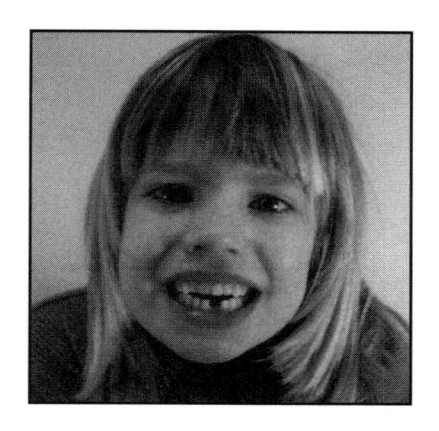

And this little piggy went wee-wee-wee all the way home.

Bare teeth and tap them as if they were chattering.

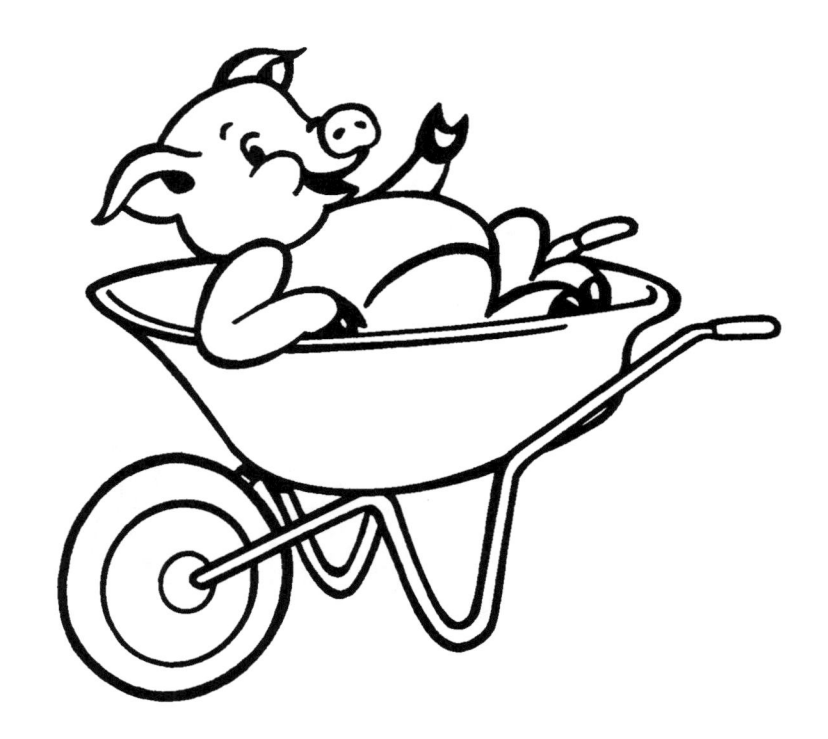

Stamp Licking

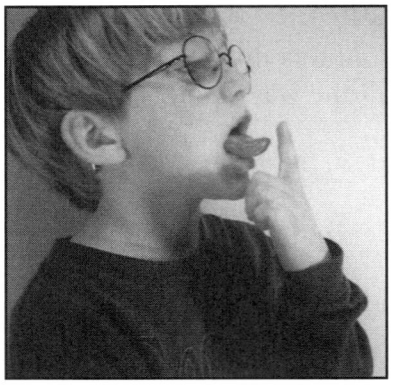

Licky-licky-licky, lick.

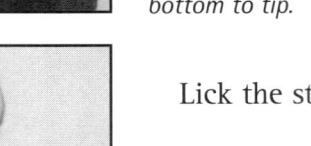

Hold out index finger and pretend to lick it from bottom to tip.

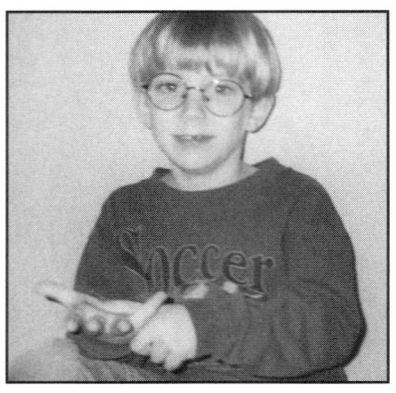

Lick the stamp to make it stick.

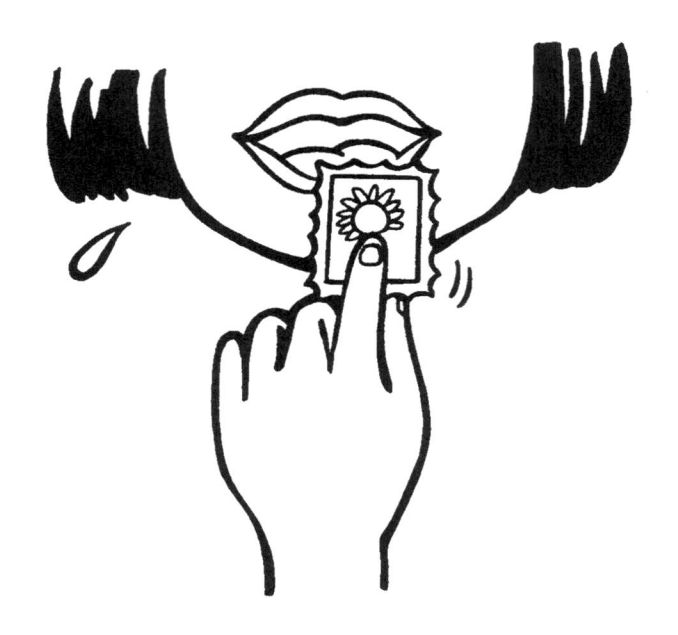

Slap your licked finger onto your opposite palm.

Zip It!

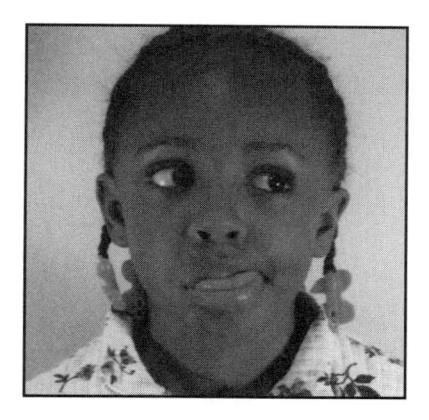

Blah-blah-blah-blah!
Blah-blah-blah-blah!
Blah-blah-blah-blah!
Blah-blah-blah-blah!
Zip it!

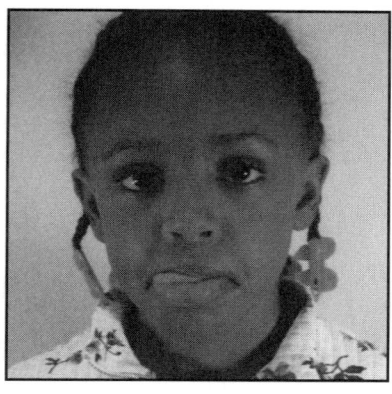

Move tongue across lips left to right and close mouth. Mime trying to talk with mouth closed. Move tongue across lips right to left and open mouth. Give a sigh of relief.

Blah-blah-blah-blah!
Blah-blah-blah-blah!
Blah-blah-blah-blah!
Blah-blah-blah-blah!
Button it!

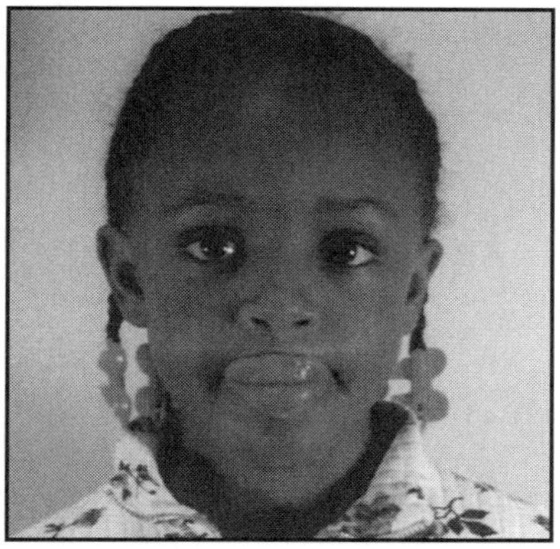

Place tongue on top lip and close mouth with tongue remaining on top lip. Mime trying to talk with mouth and tongue in this position. Move tongue away from lip and give an open-mouth sign of relief.

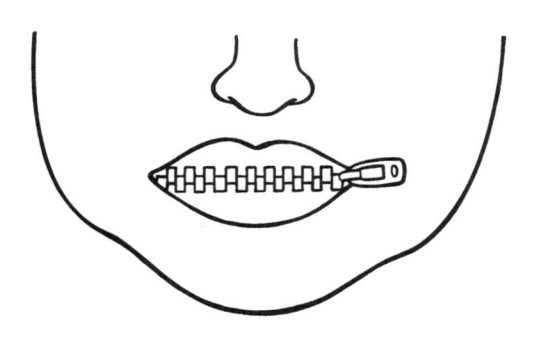

Blah-blah-blah-blah-blah!

Mouth Games

About the Mouth Games

The mouth games in this section are contests and short cause-effect activities. Mouth games work best when played individually or with small groups of two or three children. A few of the games can be set up as play center activities. Within small group settings, you can carefully guide the play and improvise motivating factors ("Blow harder!"; "Let's do it backward now!").

In mouth games, the children move objects by blowing or with mouth manipulation. The games are organized according to which mouth action is used. Materials are simple, inexpensive, and include such things as table-tennis balls and empty plastic soda bottles. Material needs are listed with each game.

Playing mouth games provides practice in moving the mouth in novel ways and motor planning new movements. The games focus the child's attention on the goal of the movement. The children can see their progress or success in the task.

Straws

Many mouth games are played by blowing or sucking through a straw. Select straws based on the type of activity and the children's oral motor capabilities.

Straws have different opening widths. The most common widths range from ⅛-inch to ¼-inch across. Buy straws made of lightweight plastic; or purchase clear plastic tubing and cut it to drinking-straw length. Tubing is more durable and can be washed, sterilized, and reused. For infection control, label the straw assigned to each child. If possible, use a different-colored straw for each child; or tag the straws, using file-folder labels or the sticky portion of low-adhesive notepad papers. Write the child's name on the label and wrap it around the straw.

Straw selection for children with specific oral motor challenges will depend on a balance between lip control and breath control. Children who have difficulty with lip closure will find it easier to form a seal with their lips around the top of wide straws. To determine the suitable sizes, observe the chldren as they drink through straws. Look for dribbling around the mouth, and observe how far the child places the straw into the mouth. Children with poor lip closure compensate by placing the straw farther back in the mouth so a seal can be formed using the tongue rather than the lips. If you notice this strategy, the child may have more success using a wider straw.

Although a larger opening allows easier lip closure, the air stream from a wider straw is more diffuse. A greater lung capacity will be required to fill the straw and create a sustained air stream. More forceful breaths will be needed for a stronger air stream. Find a compromise between the best width for lip closure and the best width for air volume. In general, straws more than $\frac{1}{4}$-inch wide are challenging in terms of air volume for children in blowing activities.

Blowing

Blow Me Over

Materials

6 to 10 sheets of construction paper in different colors

Scissors

Preparation

Cut the construction paper in 2 x 5½-inch strips. Fold the strips across the 5½-inch length and stand them in a row.

Playing the Game

This simple activity lends itself to many games.

Ask the children to blow down the papers.

See who can blow the most papers over with one breath.

Alternate colors, and ask the children to direct their air stream carefully to blow over only one color and not the others.

Line the papers in a row and blow them down like dominoes.

Vary the paper sizes.

Paper strip tents low to the floor will be harder to topple, but they can scoot! Race the papers.

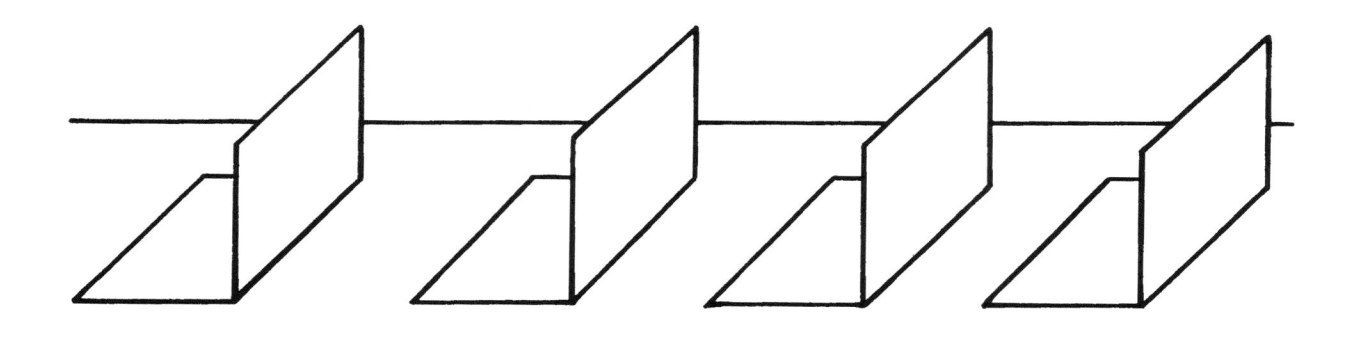

Bottle o' Bubbles

This easy game provides immediate results!

Materials

6 empty 16-ounce plastic soda bottles

Razor knife

Scissors

6 tablespoons water-soluble paint, six colors

6 teaspoons dishwashing detergent

6 cups of water

Dishpan

12-inch straws (one for each child)

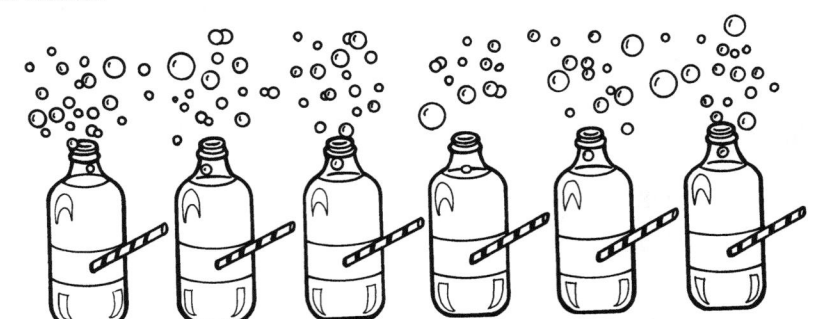

Preparation

Remove the cap from each bottle. Place each empty bottle on its side. Use the razor knife to slice a ½-inch line about halfway down the belly of the bottle. (Cut with the razor held horizontal to the table. Do not attempt to punch a hole with the razor in a vertical position above the bottle because the razor may slip, increasing the risk of injury.) Insert scissors into the cut line and cut a hole big enough for a straw. Repeat this process with the other bottles. Pour one tablespoon of paint into each bottle, one color per bottle. Add one teaspoon of detergent to each bottle. Swish the detergent and paint inside each bottle to mix. Add one cup of water to each bottle.

Playing the Game

Place the bottles in the dishpan. Give each child a straw. Tell the children to place their straws into the holes on the sides of the bubble pop bottles and blow. Lightly tinted soap bubbles will foam out of the tops of the bottles. Encourage the children to fill the dishpan with bubbles.

Variations

Adapt this game to an activity center for independent exploration. Label cups with each child's name. Store each child's straw in a cup; or provide a fresh straw each time a child approaches the center.

Choose colors to match the topic of the week.

Use a pan with high edges, and challenge the children to fill it to the top.

Try different sized plastic bottles.

Cut several straw holes in larger bottles.

Cotton Ball Clear-Out

This is a good game for success for children who cannot direct their air stream efficiently. A general puff is all that is needed to send the cotton balls scurrying.

If the children cannot resist using their hands to clear the table, give them an object to hold with two hands behind their backs.

Avoid playing this game during cold and flu season.

Materials

Bag of cotton balls

Table

Playing the Game

Place the children standing or kneeling on one side of a table, 2 feet apart from one another. (Placing the children in a row 2 feet apart distances them from each other's air stream.) Empty a bag of cotton balls onto the table. Tell the children to blow and clear the table.

Follow this game with a cotton-ball pick-up, and play again.

Variations

Create teams, placing the cotton balls on more than one table top, with one team per table; or have a race with one person per table.

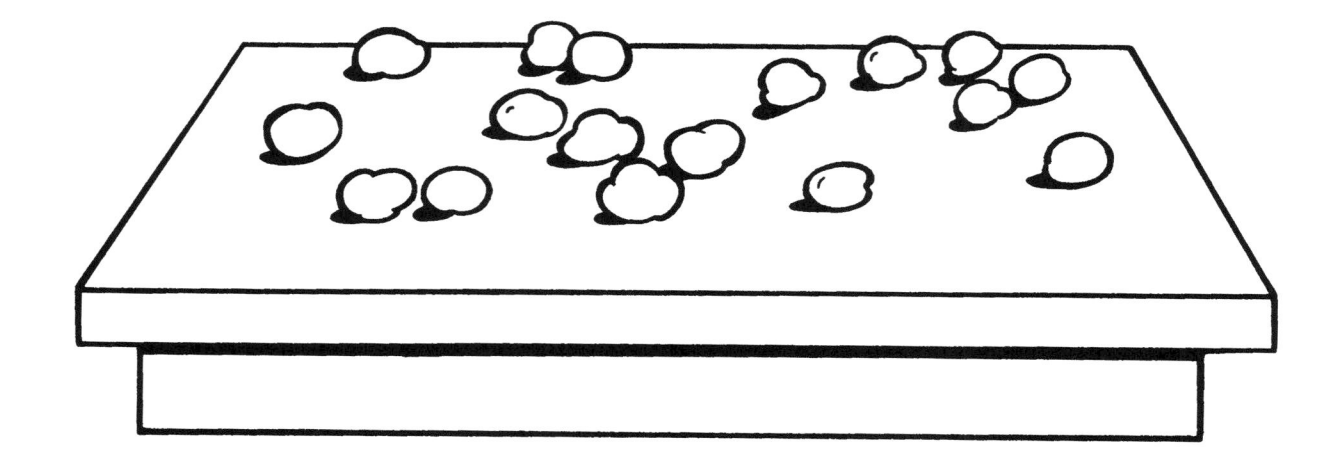

Firefighters

Play this game outdoors.

The game is not recommended for children who exhibit inappropriate spitting behaviors.

Materials

8 to 10 paper cups (Red is best, to symbolize fire)

Scissors

Railing (or board)

Paper cups (one cup for each child)

Water

Preparation

Cut the rims of several paper cups to create jagged edges that look like flames. Set the cups in a row on a railing (or create a railing by placing a board across playground equipment). Mark a boundary line 12 to 18 inches from the railing.

Playing the Game

Give each child an uncut paper cup filled with water. Tell the children, "Hold the water in your mouth, and then spit the water out in a stream to knock down the red cups and 'put out the fire.'"

Variations

The children may work cooperatively to knock down all the cups through consecutive turns.

They may compete to see how many fire cups a single child can dispatch with one cupful of water.

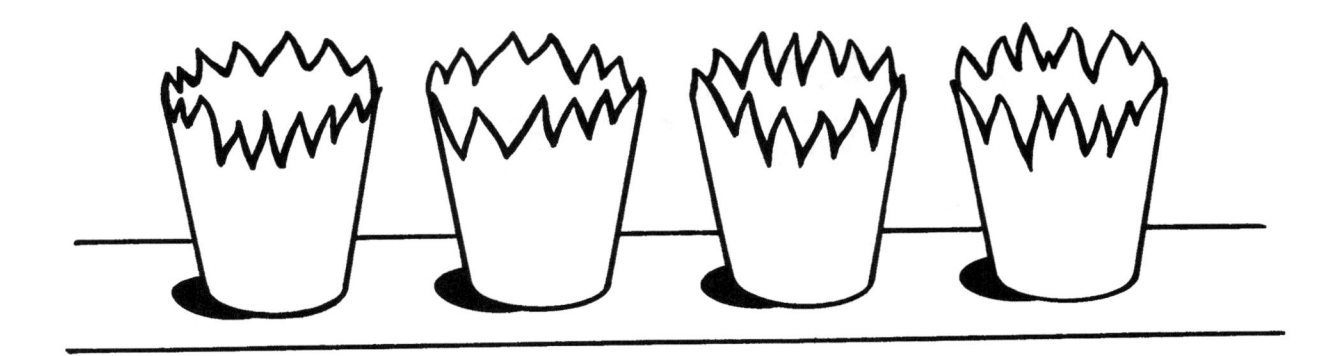

Glitter Blow

Select drawing paper according to the project.

Integrate the game with Christmas or other glitter-art projects.

Materials

Length of butcher paper (about 3 square feet for each child)

Drawing paper (one sheet for each child)

Tape

Glitter

Glue

Playing the Game

Play this game outside when it is not too windy. If doing the activity inside, tape butcher paper to the floor to collect the glitter that is not used.

Draw a shape or design with glue on the drawing paper. Place a pile of glitter on the drawing paper. Tell the children to blow the glitter until it covers the glue and reveals the shape.

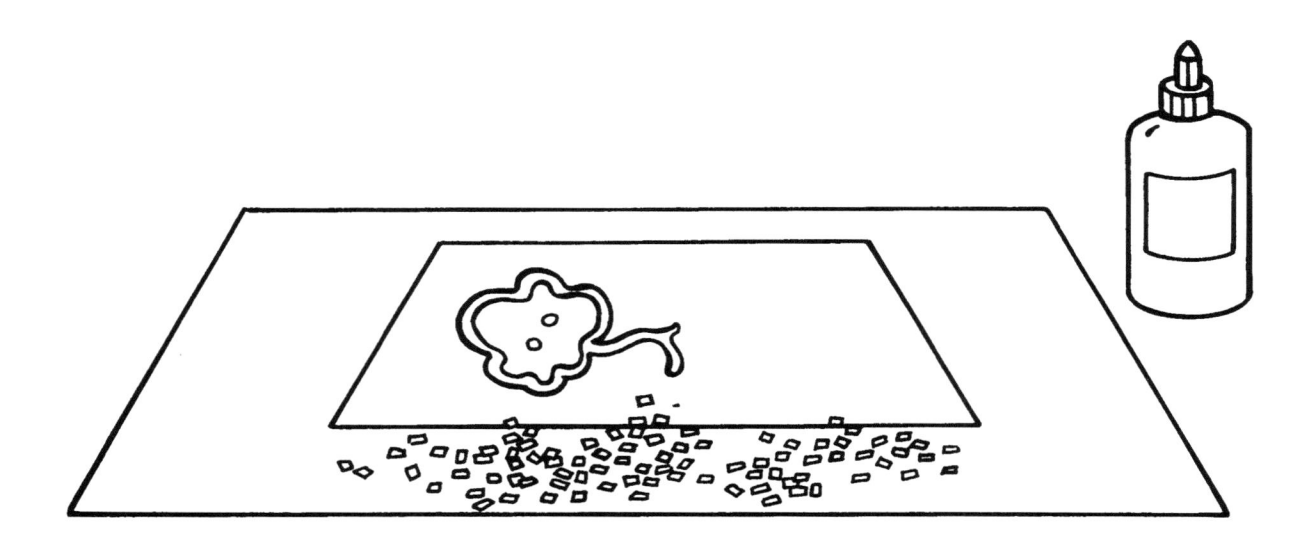

Floating Cups

Initiate this activity by demonstrating it for the children. Success requires a strong and directed air stream. The task can be made easier by filling the bottom cup with more water so the top cup sits high. Then challenge the children by gradually reducing the amount of water. The children will be motivated as they watch the top cup rise inside the bottom cup. Assist the children by participating in the blowing as needed.

Materials

2 smooth-sided light plastic cylindrical drinking cups of the same size without handles

Water

Preparation

Fill one cup one-fourth to halfway with water. Place the second cup inside the first cup. Turn the upper cup around a few times inside the bottom cup to distribute moisture. The inner cup will sit up on the water, creating a space between the two cups.

Playing the Game

Tell the children to blow into the space between the two cups. The top cup will lift up from the bottom cup. A strong air stream will lift it out completely.

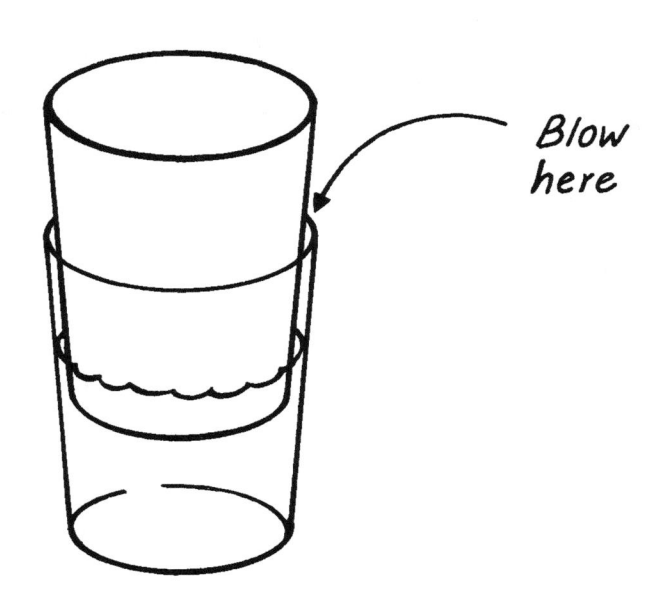

Party-Favor Ball Race

Materials

Table-tennis balls (one for each child)

Party-favor blowers (one for each child)

Chalk

Playing the Game

Give each child a party-favor blower and a table-tennis ball. Use chalk to mark START and FINISH lines on the floor. Have the children line up on hands and knees behind the START line. Tell them to place their table-tennis balls on the START line and put their party blowers in their mouths. Show the children how to move the balls by blowing through the party blowers. Say, "GO!" Using their blowers, the children push the balls across the FINISH line.

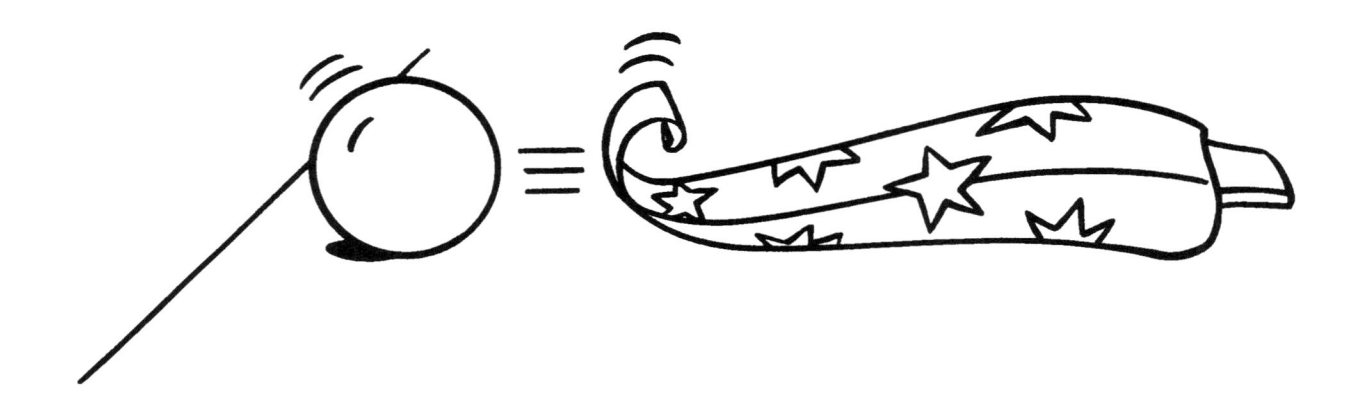

Pinwheels

Make pinwheels as a class project. Encourage the children to color a design on the paper before making the pinwheel.

Materials

- 8-inch square of paper
- Crayons
- Scissors
- 12-inch straw or dowel
- Tack or pin

Making the Pinwheels

1. Cut the square of paper diagonally, beginning at each corner and cutting toward the center. Do not cut across the center.

2. See illustration 2. Bend each marked corner to the center.

   Attach the corners to the center, using a pin.

3. Pin the center to a dowel or straw.

   Blow the pinwheel.

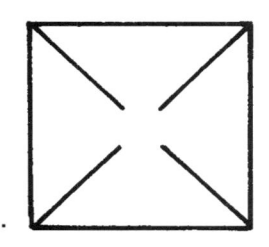

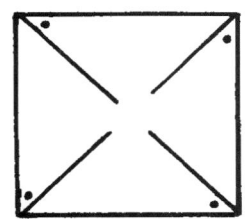

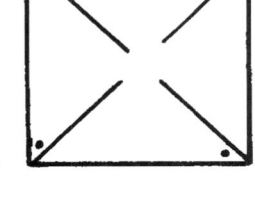

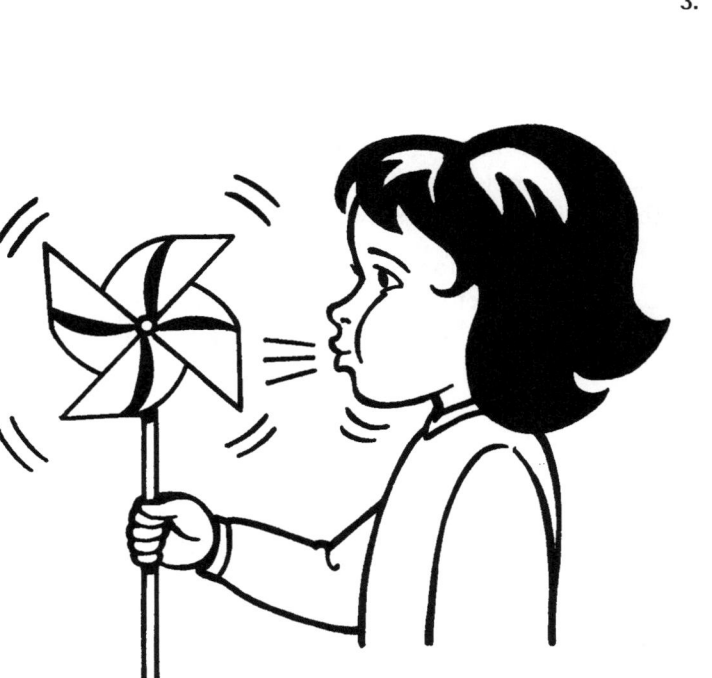

Playing-Card People

Materials

Playing cards with pictures (one card for each player)

Old, disposable playing cards (or lightweight index cards and scissors)

Paper clips

Colored masking tape

Table

Preparation

Select playing cards with pictures—children's cards with animals or other figures, or the king, queen, and jack from a standard deck. Match each picture card with a disposable card. If you do not have any old, disposable cards, cut index cards into playing-card size.

1. Fold the card in half.

2. Lift one edge to make another fold ½-inch from the folded edge. Turn the card over and repeat on the other side. Grasp the original fold and place the card on the table. (See illustration 2.)

3. The two ends will extend from a raised fold in the middle. (See illustration 3.)

4. Clip the picture card to this raised fold. Now the picture card is standing up.

Playing the Game

Use colored masking tape to mark a circle on the top of a table. Show the children how to blow their cards so they arrive in the center circle. The cards move along the table as if the playing-card people were walking.

The objective in this activity is for the playing-card people to stay upright. Younger children may prefer to send their playing-card people running across the table to fall down on the other side.

Variations

Set up different targets as different rooms. Challenge the children to send their people into certain rooms on one breath, without toppling the playing-card person over the edge of the table.

Have the children race their people across the table.

Blowing harder on one side of the card will make it spin around. Have the playing-card people dance.

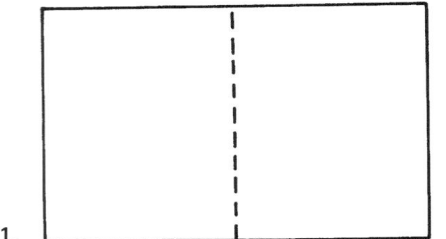

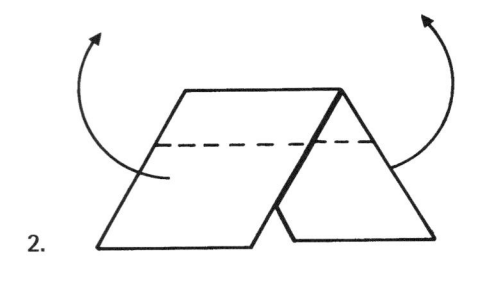

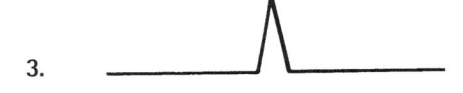

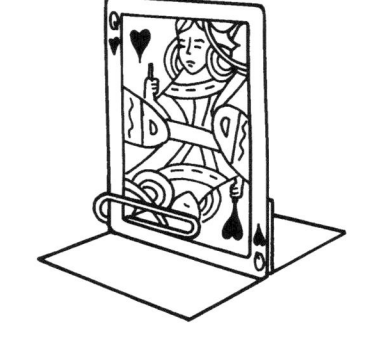

Blowing Down the Road

In this activity, the children must focus and redirect their airflow to maneuver the curves. For very young children, a straight distance of one foot is sufficient. Although a table-tennis ball weighs very little, children who have difficulty directing their air stream with efficiency will have difficulty moving the ball with their breath.

Materials

Table-tennis balls (one for each child)

Yarn

Scissors

Playing the Game

Using yarn, lay out a curving "road" with two yarn "curbs" for the ball to roll between. Have the first child get down on hands and knees at the beginning of the road. Place a ball in front of the child. Tell the child to blow the ball down the road.

Variations

As control improves, use different grades of ball types. Plastic foam balls are easy to move, but difficult to control. Balls made of light foam move more easily than table-tennis balls and have sufficient weight for control of direction. To challenge children with good breath control, use heavier balls of solid plastic.

Increase the distance and number of curves in the road as the children acquire skill.

Lay out several roads for races.

Make a town of roads for play.

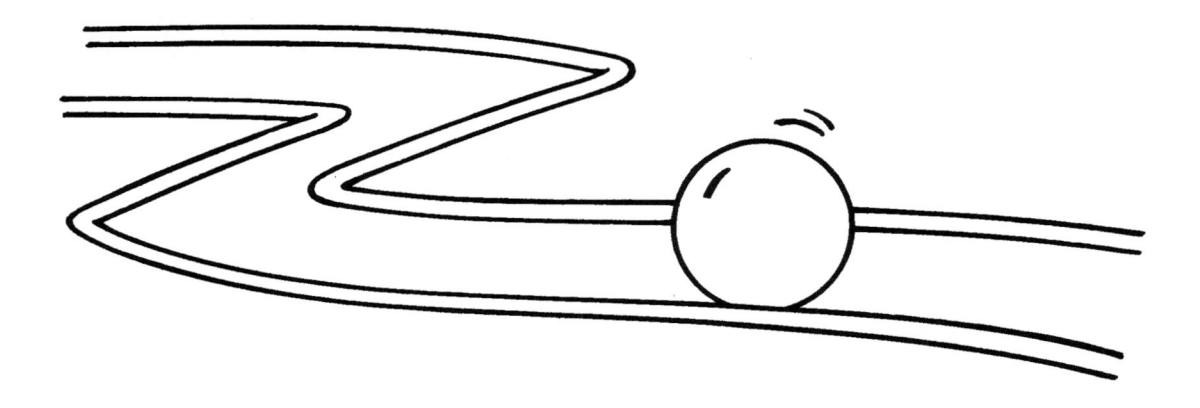

Pooh!

Introduce this game by demonstrating it for the children. Blow the tissue hard so it flies straight up. The children are usually delighted to see this and anxious to try it themselves.

Materials

Facial tissues (one for each child)

Playing the Game

Have the children lie on their backs. Place a facial tissue over each child's face. Tell the children to blow hard. A strong, directed air stream will lift the tissue off their faces.

Very young children will have difficulty blowing hard with a narrow enough air stream to make the tissue fly. Give them opportunity to practice.

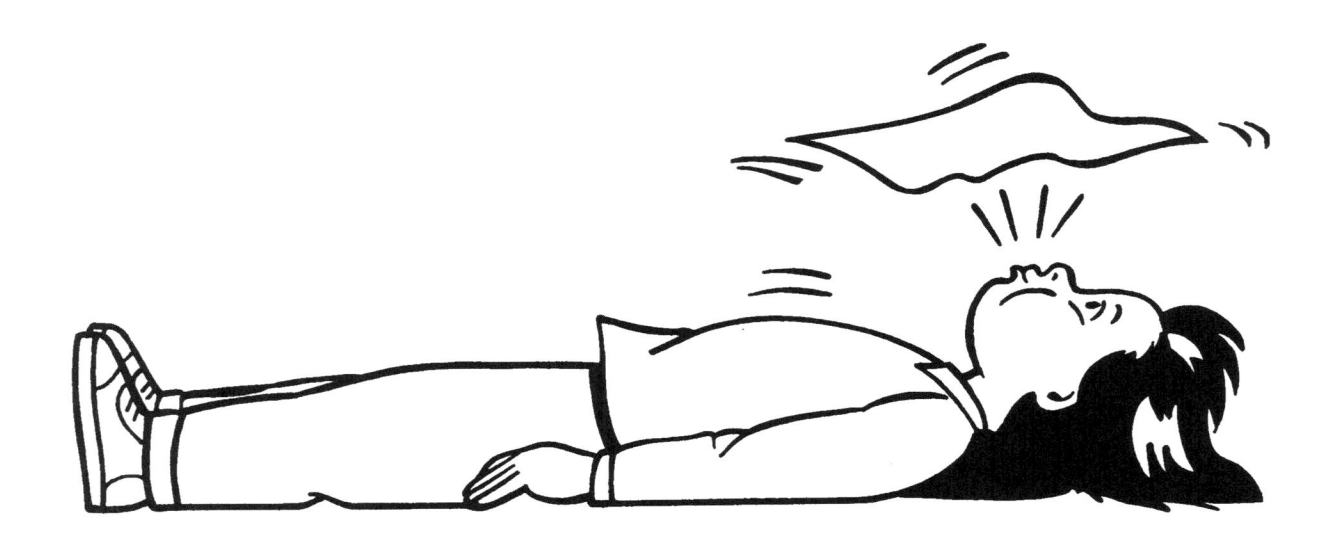

Pucker Power

This game is only as difficult as the toys you select. Experiment with several lightweight toys. Place the toys on a flat surface and see how hard it is to blow them over.

If the children cannot imitate the pucker "pah," allow them to simply blow.

Materials

Lightweight toys

Table

Playing the Game

Set up the chosen toys in a row on a table. Show the children how to gather air in their mouths, filling their cheeks. Then have them release the air all at once in a "pah," toppling the toys.

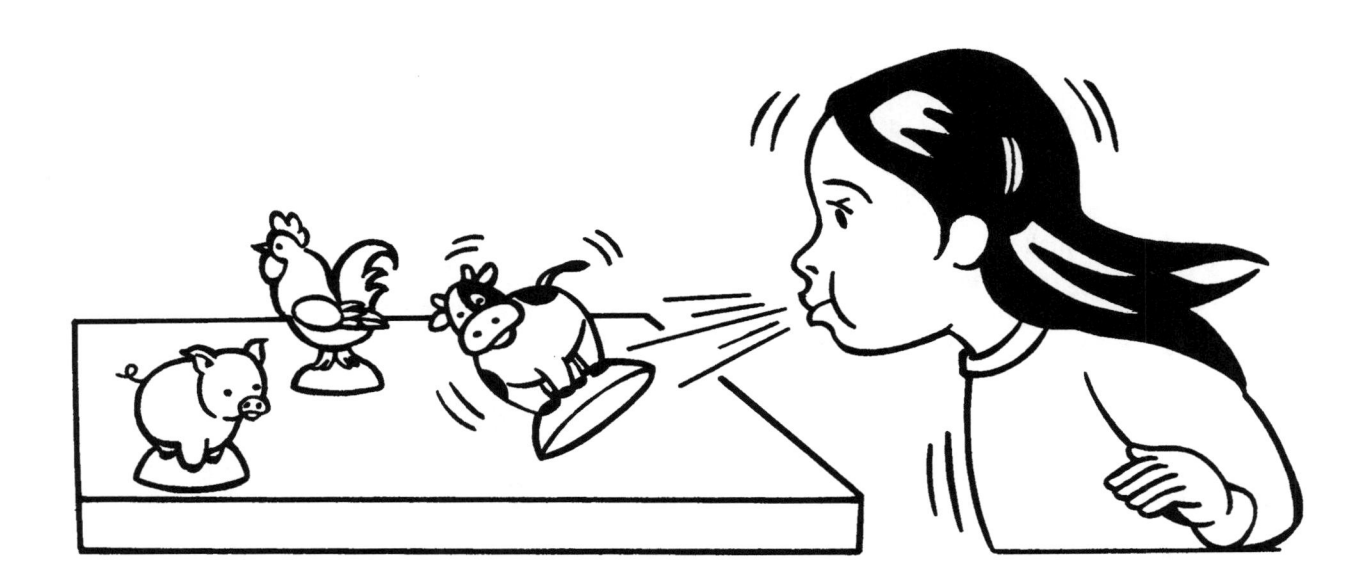

Rattle Blow

Materials

Empty 16-ounce plastic soda bottles (one for each child)

Razor knife

Scissors

Scraps of colored paper

Preparation

Remove the cap from each bottle. Place each empty bottle on its side. Use the razor knife to slice a ½-inch line about 2 inches from the bottom of the bottle. (Cut with the razor knife held horizontal to the table. Do not attempt to punch a hole with the razor in a vertical position above the bottle because the razor may slip, increasing the risk of injury.) Insert scissors into the cut line and cut a hole about ¼- to ½-inch in diameter. Repeat this process with the other bottles.

Playing the Game

Tell the children to tear the scraps of paper into very small pieces, about 1 inch in diameter, and to wad them up into little balls. Have the children poke these little paper balls into their bottles. Show them how to blow into the tops of their bottles to make the paper balls fly and swirl.

Hints

Be sure to cut holes no larger than ½-inch square in the bottles; larger holes will make it more difficult to fill the bottle with air. Prompt the children to place their lips *within* rather than *over* the top of the bottle end when blowing. It is more difficult to create a strong air stream in a wide-open mouth position. A strong blow may flip a paper ball out of the bottle blow hole, which usually adds to the children's excitement.

Variations

Use different weights of paper.

Vary the color of the paper. Moisture from the children's breath will cloud the sides of the bottle, so darker-colored paper is most effective.

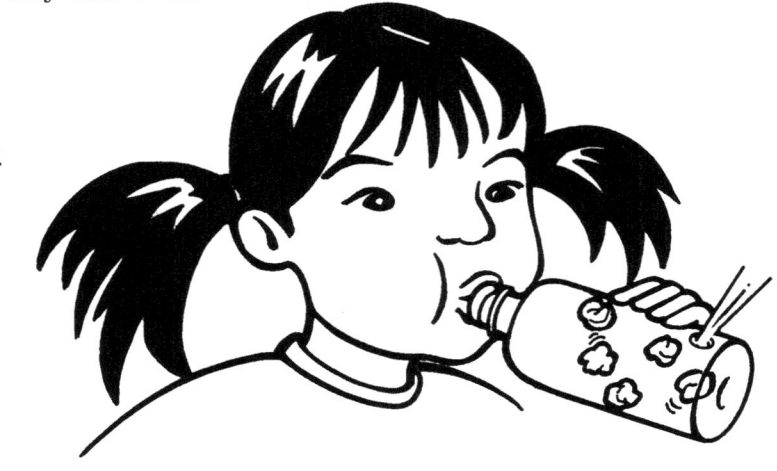

Visual and Kinesthetic Whistles

Next time you go shopping, think about the oral motor challenges that a whistle can provide. Look in toy and party shops for whistles that do more than make noise. These whistles are available in a wide variety—bubble pipes, kazoos, warbling-bird water whistles, whistles that send a thread spinning, and others.

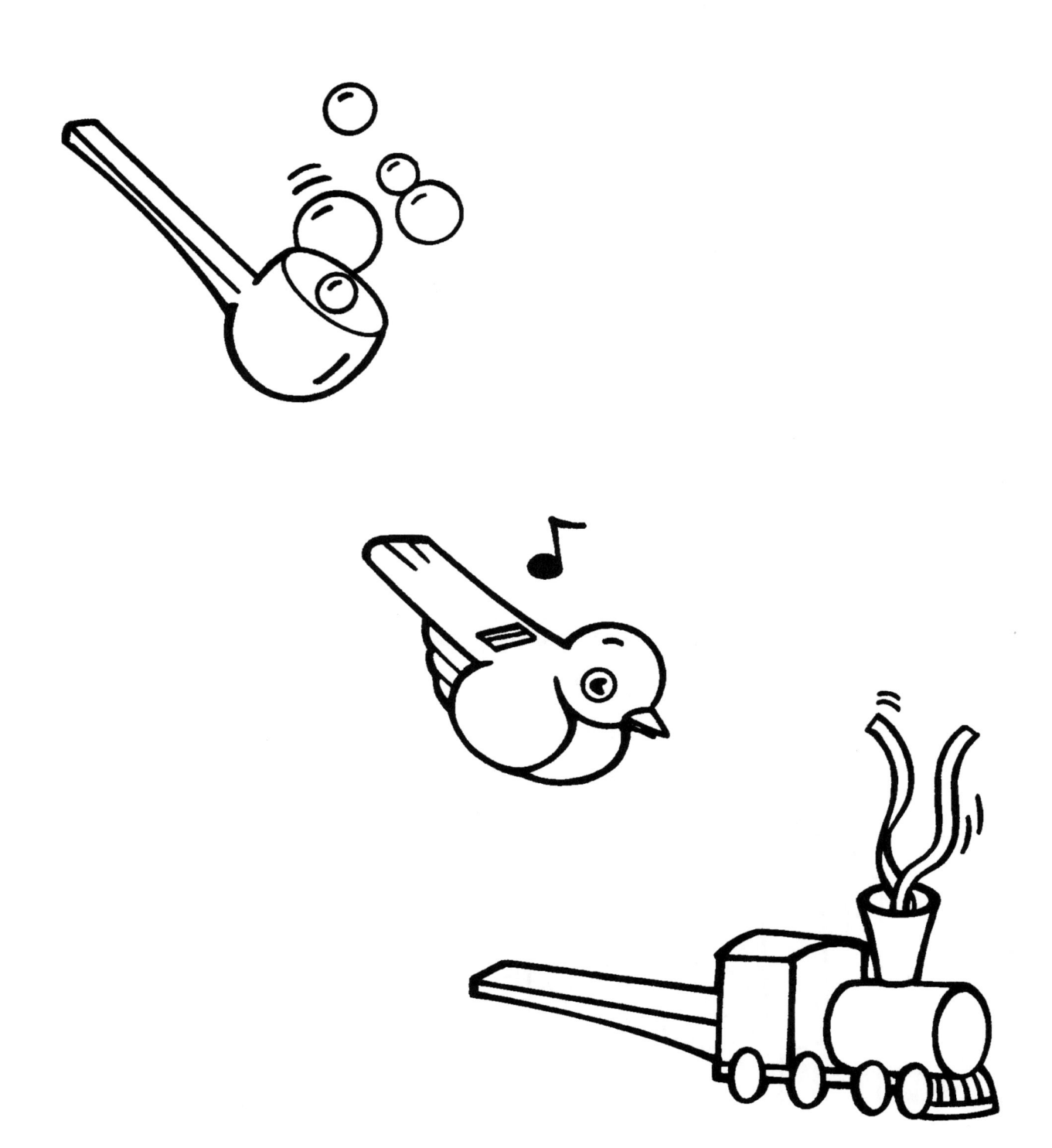

Water Table Boats

Materials

Empty ½-pint cardboard milk cartons (one for each boat)

Scissors

Craft sticks (one for each boat)

Tape

Paper

Water table (or shallow tub filled with water)

Preparation

Rinse the milk cartons and let them dry. Cut each milk carton in half. Discard the top half. Make the mast by taping a craft stick inside the front of the carton. To make the sail, cut a 4-inch square of paper. Cut two ½-inch slits about 2 inches apart in the center of the paper, and thread the craft stick through these two holes to make the sail.

Playing the Game

Place the boats in the water table (or fill a shallow tub with water and place the boats in the tub). Tell the children to blow the boats. The lightweight boats move easily across the water.

Make extra sails to replace wet ones.

Variations

Encourage the children to experiment with their blows. Strong blows will topple the boats. Gentle blows will sail them. Blowing high or low also will have different effects. Talk about the weather.

Encourage the children to have boat races.

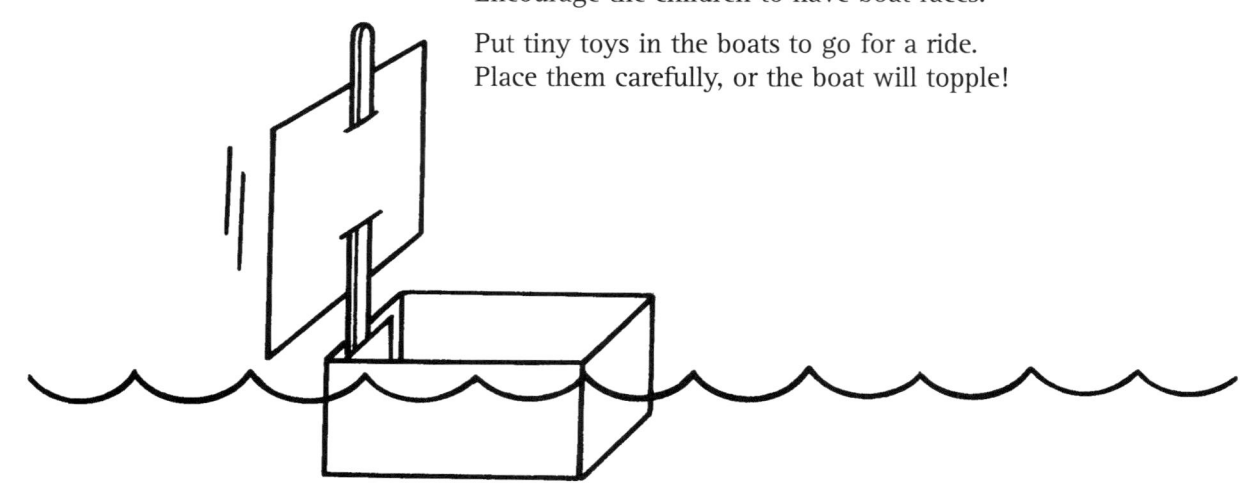

Put tiny toys in the boats to go for a ride. Place them carefully, or the boat will topple!

Manipulating

Crayon Mouth Sticks

Materials

Fat crayons (one for each child)

Paper towels (one for each child)

Playing the Game

Fold the paper towel into a small square slightly larger than the child's mouth. Fold the towel square over the end of a large crayon. Show the children how to hold the crayon in the mouth by gently biting over the folded paper towel and the crayon's end inside. Ask the children to draw with their mouths. This is not a simple task. Begin by having the children draw straight lines. As skills improve, challenge them to color small pictures, trace lines, or write their names using their mouth.

The paper towel disperses the pressure needed to hold the crayon end steady and absorbs saliva.

Variations

Draw a road on a piece of paper, and have the children follow it with their crayons. As the children have success with this task, add twists and turns to the road.

Rinse the crayons carefully before permitting the children to trade crayons.

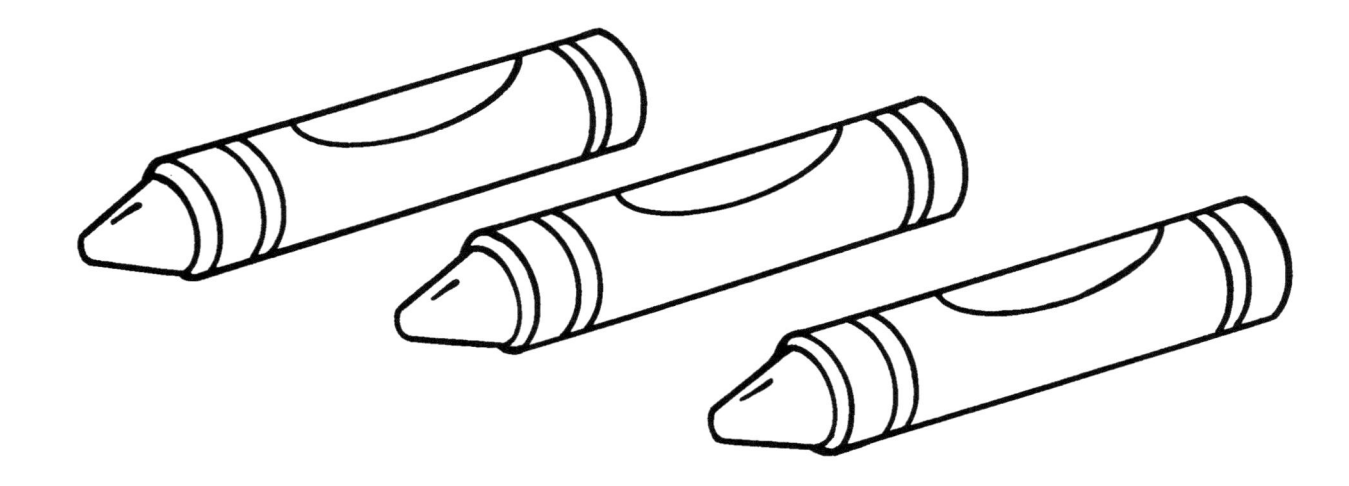

Mister Chin Man

Materials

Water-soluble eyebrow pencil

Pillows (one for each child)

Hand mirror

Yarn (optional)

Bow ties (optional)

Playing the Game

Use the eyebrow pencil to draw two eyes and a nose on each child's chin. Orient the drawing upside down so the "nose" is directly under the child's mouth and the "eyes" are near the child's jaw line. Position the children in pairs back-to-back or in a small circle, backs to the center. Have the children lie down, and place a pillow under each child's shoulders. Tell the children to tilt their heads back, look at each other's chins, and talk. ("Hello! I'm Mister Chin Man!") Have Mister Chin Man say his vowels.

Very young children do not visualize Mister Chin Man easily. Be distinct when drawing the nose and eyes. Pass a hand mirror around the circle, so the children can see themselves being Mister Chin Man. You may want to add yarn hair or a bow tie.

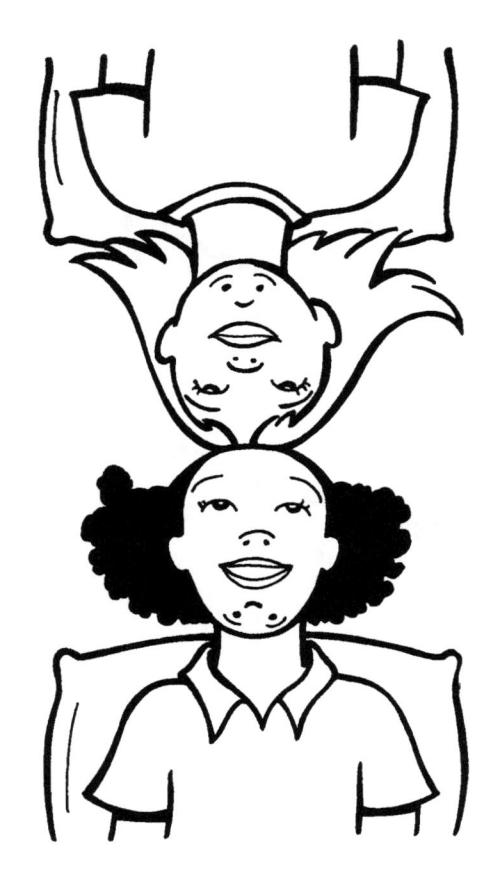

Kissing Pictures

Materials

- Cotton-tipped swabs
- Lipstick
- Facial tissues
- Paper plates, coffee filters, construction paper, or other surfaces

Playing the Game

Using a fresh cotton-tipped swab for each child, apply lipstick generously to the children's lips. Have them kiss paper plates or other surfaces. Send the kissing pictures home to Mom and Dad.

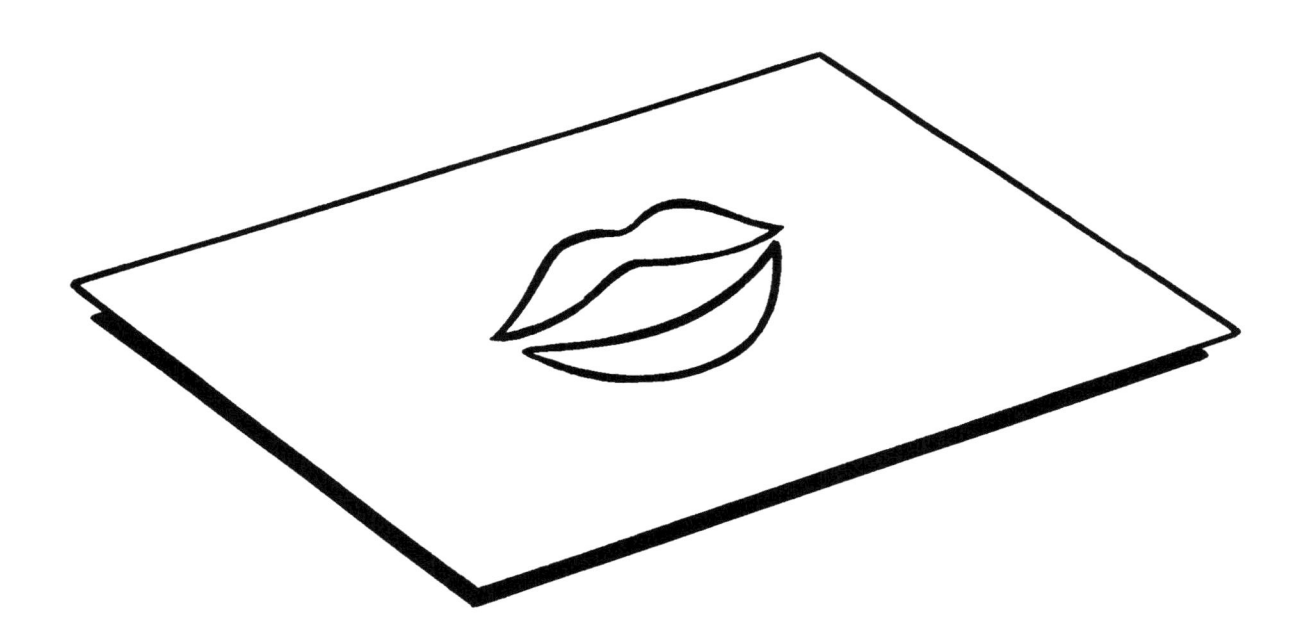

Mustache Trick

Materials

Unsharpened pencils (one for each child)

Playing the Game

Tell the children to place the pencil lengthwise between their lip and nose. Show them how to curl the upper lip and hold the pencil with their lip and not their hands.

For an advanced trick, have the children move the pencil from the upper lip into the mouth without using their hands.

1. Be sure the lip is holding the pencil at the midpoint of its length.

2. Tilt the face up before releasing the pencil from the lip. Allow the pencil to roll naturally into the mouth.

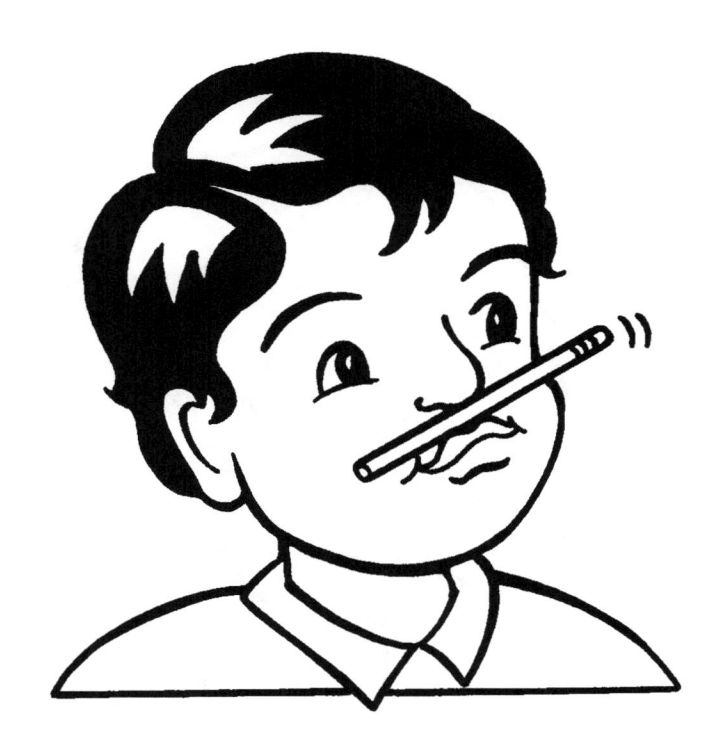

Muffle Face

Introduce this game by demonstrating it to the children. The towel-mouth effect is funny. Be sure they show each other their funny faces.

Materials

Paper towels (one for each child)

Scissors

Mirror

Crayons (optional)

Playing the Game

Cut or tear two holes for eyes in the paper towel. Have the children hold the towel masks over their faces. Tell the children to look in the mirror. Have them suck some of the towel into their mouths and talk.

To prolong the game, have the children color the towels to make different types of faces.

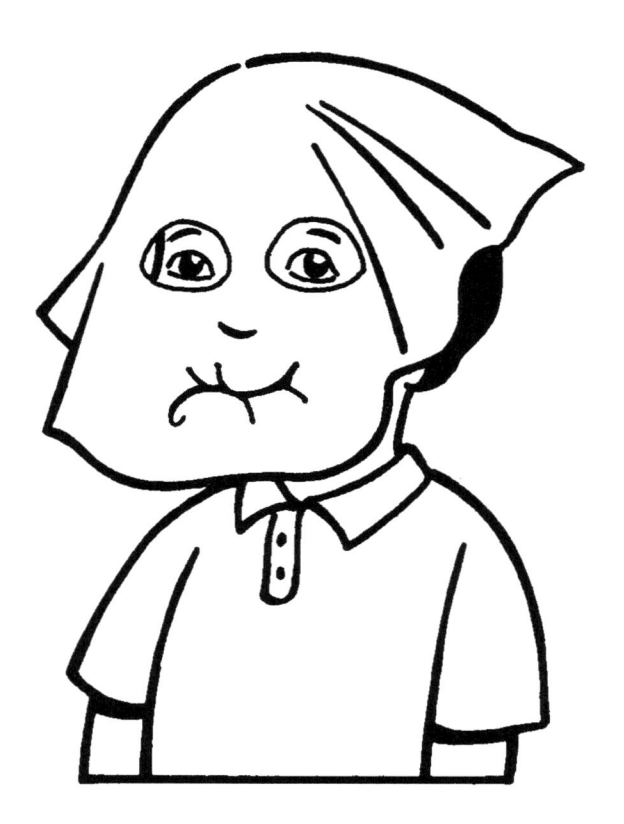

Natural Mouth Kazoos

Materials

A mirror wide enough for several children to see their faces

Playing the Game

Seat the children in front of the mirror. Show the children how to make a sustained sound. Tell them to say "Ooooo." Practice until the children can sustain the sound for about five seconds. Combine the sound with one or all of these face manipulations to create a vibratory or kazoo effect. Choose a tune with many sustained notes (such as *Taps* or *The Star Spangled Banner*), or extend and sustain the notes on other songs. Alternate face manipulations at different points in the song.

Annie's Cheek Pull—Pinch right cheek with right hand, left cheek with left hand. Pull cheeks rapidly back and forth.

Clown Grin—Put right index finger into right side of mouth, left index finger into left side of mouth. Wiggle fingers back and forth, stretching and relaxing the mouth.

Steel Guitar Sound Effect—Slightly pucker the lips. Run finger up and down the lips.

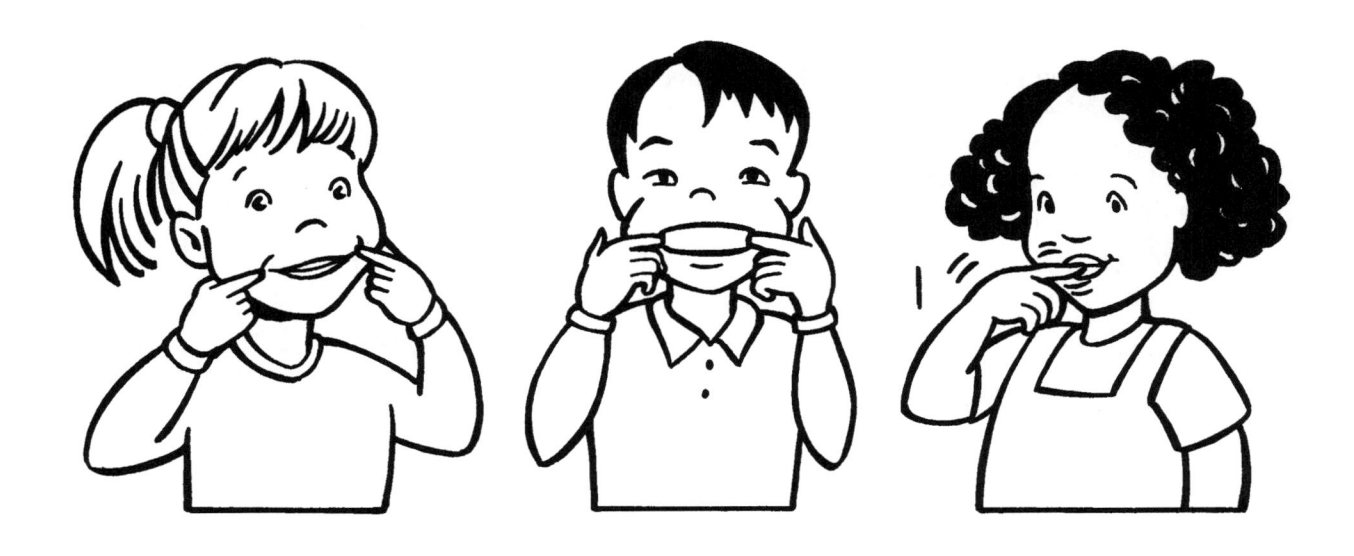

Puppy Pick-Up Sticks

This game requires the child to manipulate and hold at the same time. Children who have difficulty will use their hands to compensate. To maintain interest in mastering the game, allow this compensation for the harder parts while encouraging the children to do the trick without using their hands on the easier parts.

Materials

Stiff plastic straws or small rods (three for each child)

Playing the Game

Play this game on the floor, with the children on their hands and knees in a circle, facing inward. Give three straws to each child. Have the children lay their straws horizontally on the floor in front of them. Tell them to listen and follow the directions. Give the directions:

"Little Puppy Pick-Up Sticks picked up one stick!"—Each child bends down like a puppy, picks up one straw using only the mouth, secures the straw in the mouth, and returns to all-fours position.

"Little Puppy Pick-Up Sticks put it down!"—Each child bends down and drops the one straw.

"Little Puppy Pick-Up Sticks picked up two sticks, one at a time!"—Each child bends down like a puppy, picks up one straw using only the mouth, secures the straw in the mouth, picks up another straw, and returns to all fours position.

"He put them down one at a time!"—Each child bends down, drops one straw, and then drops the other.

"Little Puppy Pick-Up Sticks picked up three sticks, one at a time!"—Each child bends down, picks up one straw using only the mouth, secures the straw in the mouth, picks up another straw, secures the two straws, picks up a third straw, and returns to all-fours position.

"He put them down one at a time!"—Each child bends down and drops the straws one at a time.

"Good Little Puppy Pick-Up Sticks!"

Encourage the children to sit up on their knees and bark like good little puppies.

Ring Fetch

Materials

Colorful craft pipe cleaners (five for each player)

A box, approximately 4 x 8 x 11 inches

Preparation

Bend and twist the pipe cleaners into circles. Ask each child to select a ring of a different color. Twist each selected pipe cleaner ring into a figure eight. Be sure the twisted ends of the bent pipe cleaner are at the cross of the figure eight and not at the top or bottom of the figure. Curl the figure eight into a hook. Avoid collapsing the figure eight. Create rounded rather than pointed ends on the hook. Drop the remaining pipe cleaner rings into the box so that they catch on one another and do not rest flat on the bottom.

Playing the Game

Show the children how to hold their figure-eight hooks in their mouths. The mouth holds the top loop of the figure eight, while the bottom of the figure eight forms a hook. Have the children hook the rings out of the box.

Variation

Play this activity as a relay. The children pass the rings to one another on their hooks. Again, be sure to avoid a pointed end on the hook, because these hooks will be passing close to other children's faces. Be sure the sharp twisted ends of the pipe cleaner figure eight is at the cross of the hooks and thus away from the mouth or the protruding ends.

It's a Tornado!

Materials

Paper plates (one for each child)

Straws (one for each child)

Water

Nontoxic crayons (optional)

Juice or sweet drinks (optional)

Playing the Game

Give each child a paper plate and a straw. Pour a small amount of water on the plate.

Have the children pretend to be tornadoes over lakes, sucking up the water with their straws.

Variations

Encourage the children to see who can be first to finish drinking the water.

Using nontoxic crayons, draw a town on the plates. Wipe off "crayon crumbs" before adding water. Tell the children to "Save the town from the flood."

Substitute juice or favorite sweet drinks for the water.

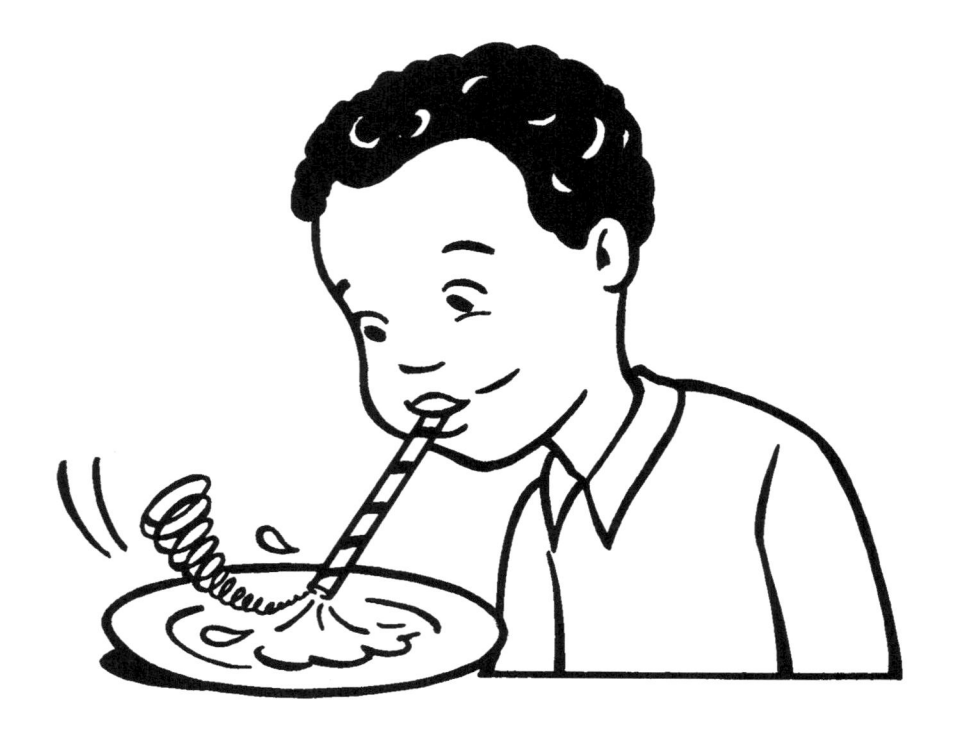

Typewriter Carriage

Materials

Stiff straws or unsharpened pencils (one for each child)

Playing the Game

Give each child a straw. Have the children position their straws horizontally between their teeth so that one end is close to the left cheek and the other end sticks farther out on the right. Show the children how to use their mouths to move the straw to the other side so the long end of the straw now protrudes from the left.

To simplify this activity, place the straw horizontally between the teeth at the midpoint of the straw. Tilt the head laterally to one side, and work on controlling the straw as it slides down. Try not to drop the straw.

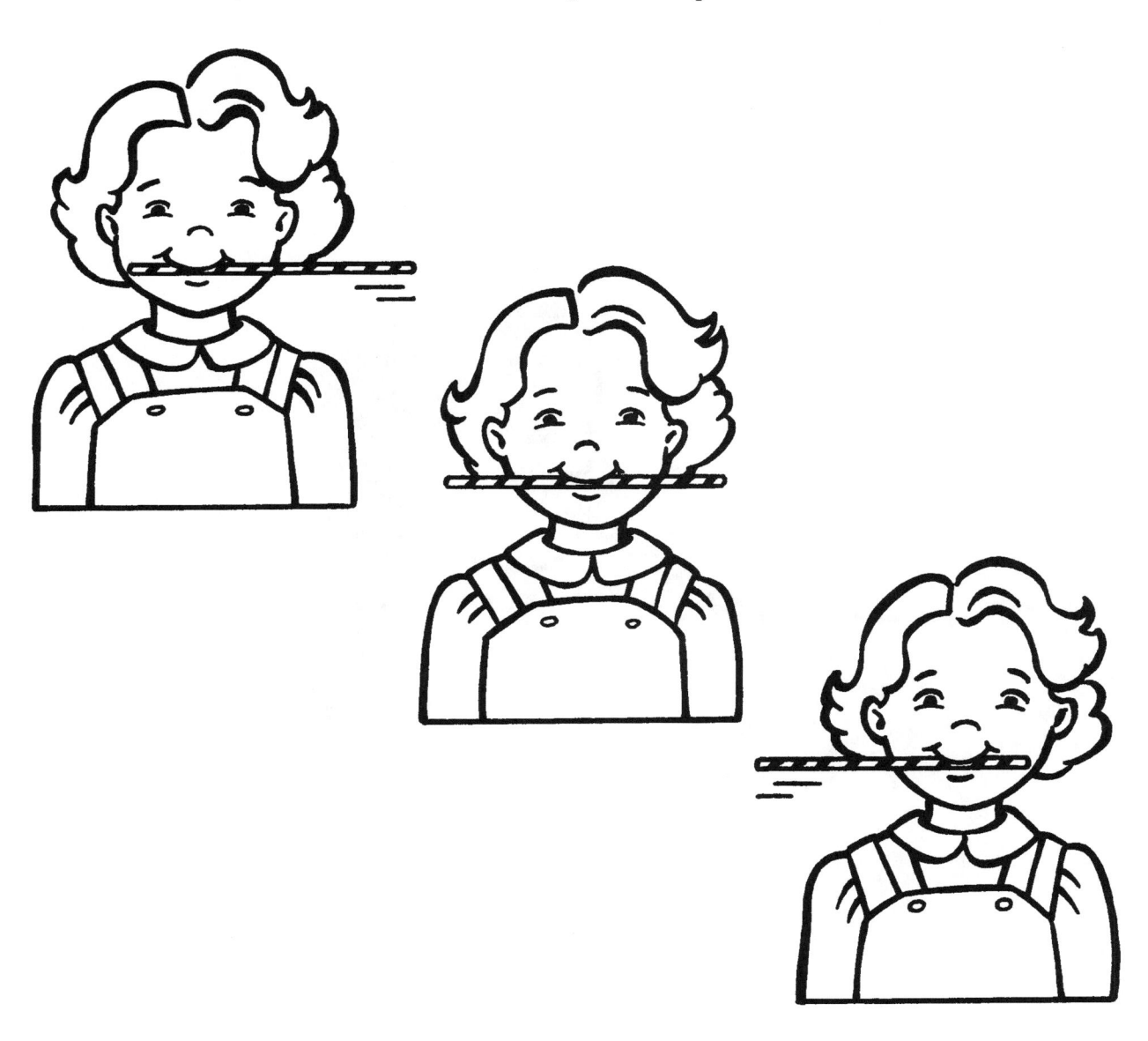

The Vacuum Cleaner

Although most children can drink from a straw, it is difficult to convey to them the need to suck rather than blow to lift the tissue. Use very lightweight paper and lots of patience!

Materials

Facial tissues (or squares of lightweight paper tissue)

Straws (one for each child)

A container

Playing the Game

Scatter the tissues in front of the children. Show the children how to put one end of the straw on the tissue and lift it by sucking through the straw. Challenge the children to lift and release all the tissues into the container.

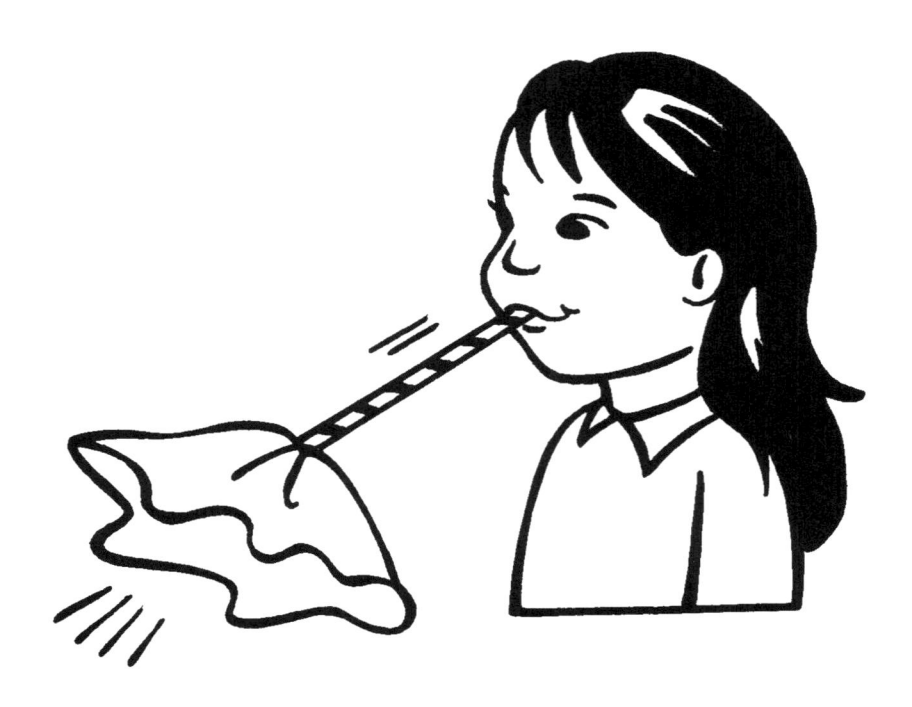

Which Way Did It Go?

Materials

Straws (one for each child)

Table-tennis ball (or stuffed animal toy)

Playing the Game

Give each child a straw. Tell the children to put their straws in their mouths. Roll a ball to the right, and ask, "Which way did it go?" Have the children shift their straws to point to the right. Repeat with different directions—left, up, down.

Variation

Substitute a stuffed animal toy for the ball. Walk the animal in different directions.

Vary the game by having the children use their straws to indicate which way they want you to move the animal.

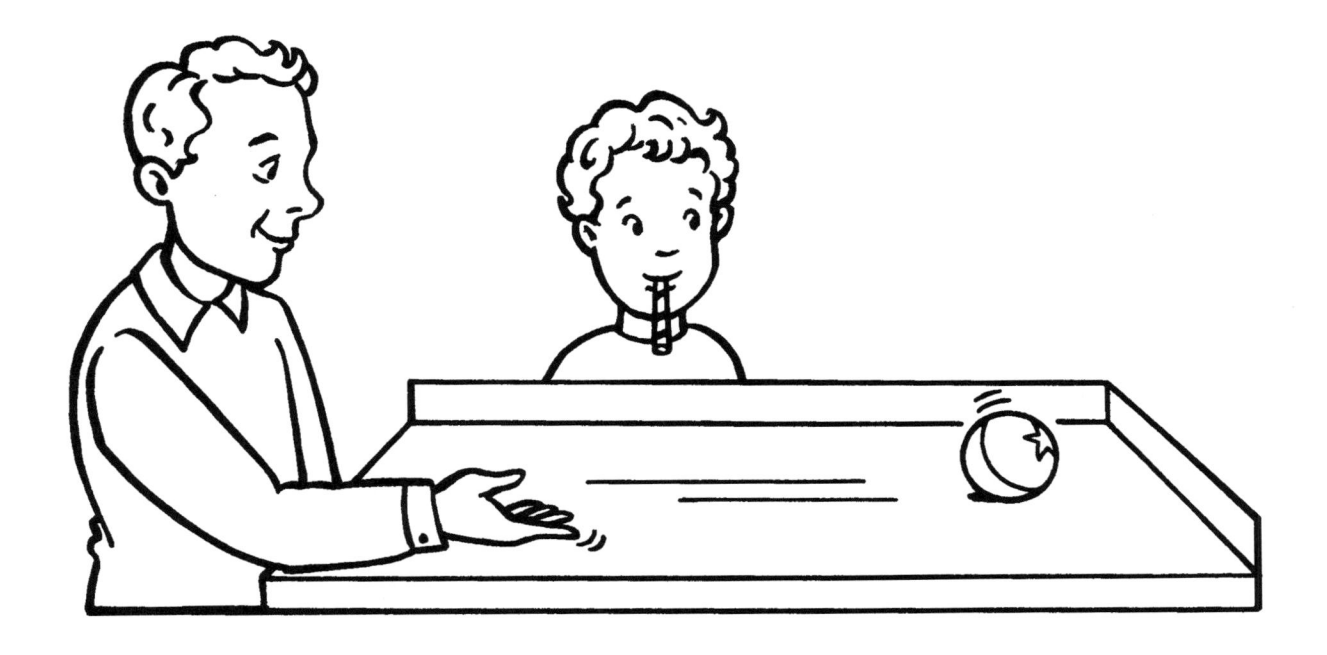

Silly Snacks

About Silly Snacks

Silly Snacks introduce funny ways to eat food. It is best to use these activities in a game context and not as part of a meal. Most of the activities involve eating without using the hands, which might be confusing for children who are trying to learn proper table manners and use of eating utensils. For children who can discriminate between appropriate mealtime and play behaviors, Silly Snacks may be appropriate at dessert time.

Silly Snacks are not recommended for children with pronounced eating difficulties. These games are designed only for children who can independently and effectively consume a standard meal. Caution is crucial when using Silly Snacks with children who have any oral motor control deficit in eating. Children with poor oral control in eating often use their hands to help move the food around in the mouth. Discouraging the use of hands, as many Silly Snacks do, increases the risk of choking for these children. Consultation with an occupational therapist or speech pathologist is needed before administering any food to children with less than optimal oral motor control. With these children, use Silly Snacks in a one-to-one situation only. Evaluate the snack for safety factors in eating method and food texture.

The foods used in Silly Snacks are typical childhood treats. They include miniature marshmallows, raisins, pudding, and breakfast cereal. Individual children's dietary restrictions must be followed when using these snack games.

Silly Snacks provide experiences with moving the mouth in new ways. Motor planning experiences are linked with the purpose of the activity. Silly Snacks create a motor planning connection between eating and new mouth movements.

Banana Shish Kebabs

Materials

Bananas (half or one for each child)

Uncooked regular (not thin) spaghetti or linguine (one strand for each child)

Paper towels (one for each child)

Eating the Snack

Seat the children at the table. Place a paper towel in front of each child. Peel the banana. Thread an uncooked spaghetti strand through the center of the banana. If the banana is too long, use only half the banana. Make a banana shish kebab for each child. Show the children how to grasp the shish kebab by holding the left end of the spaghetti strand with the left hand and the right end with the right hand. Tell the children to eat their banana kabobs. As the children eat their kabobs, banana pieces will fall onto the paper towels.

Variation

For an advanced challenge, tell the children to take tiny bites and see how long they can keep their bananas on the spaghetti strands.

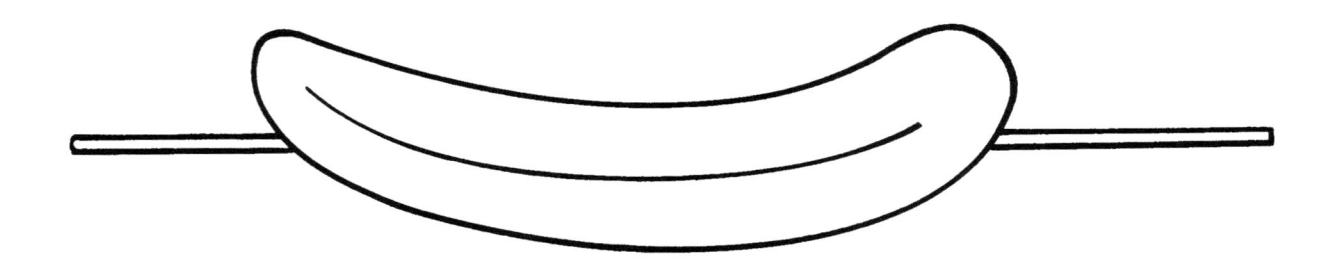

Bobbing for Grapes

Materials

Bowls, at least six inches wide (one for each child)

Grapes (one serving for each child)

Water

Eating the Snack

Seat the children at the table. Remove the grapes from the stems and place some in each bowl. Pour in enough water to cover the bottom of the bowl. Place the bowls in front of the children. Tell the children to eat their grapes without using their hands.

Adding water to the bottom of the bowl adds a slippery factor to the task. Barely cover the bottom of the bowl with water. Water over $1/8$-inch deep might end up in the children's noses as they try to trap the grapes in their mouths. The first bites will be easier, because there are more grapes to stabilize the others in the bowl. Children are likely to give up and use their hands on the last few grapes. Let the children stand up or stabilize the bowl with their hands as they chase the grapes.

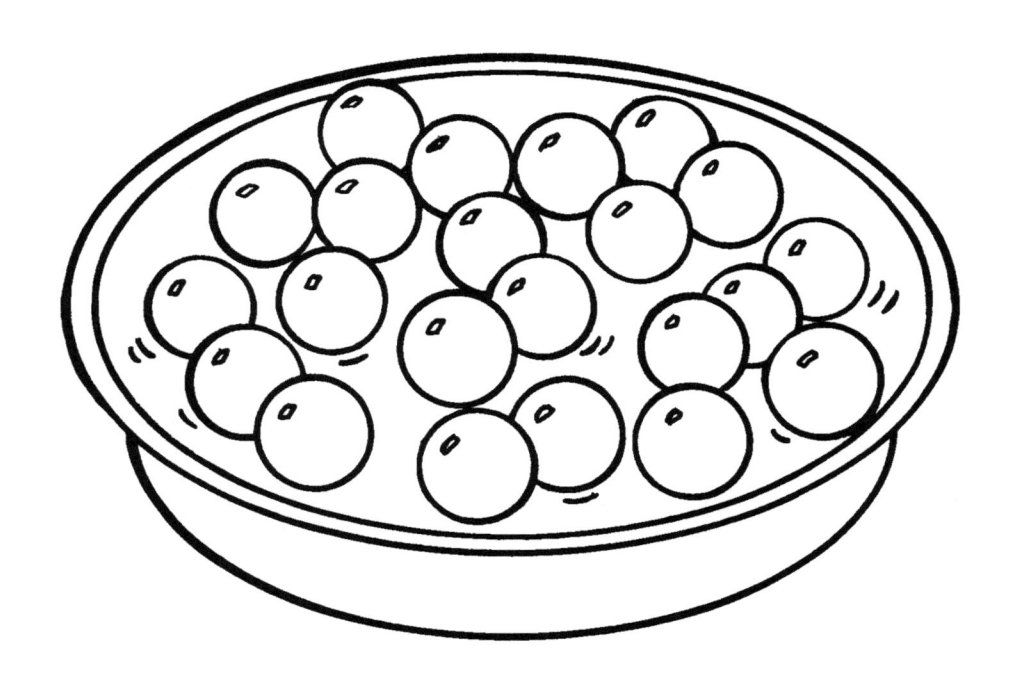

Caramel Puffed Plates

Materials

    Caramel (two pieces for each child)

    Microwaveable bowl

    Water

    Microwave oven

    Paper plates (one for each child)

    Puffed cereal (one serving for each child)

    String (one short length for each paper plate)

    Paper towels and water for cleanup

Preparation

Place the caramel pieces in the microwaveable bowl. Add one teaspoon of water for every two pieces. Microwave 20 seconds at a time, stirring between heatings, until the caramel is melted. Dribble the caramel onto the paper plates. Drop puffed cereal onto the hot caramel so that it sticks to the plate. Let the caramel cool. Punch two holes horizontal to one another, 4 inches apart across the top $1/3$ of each paper plate. Thread the string through the holes, and hang the plates against the wall or a bulletin board at each child's mouth level.

Eating the Snack

Tell the children to eat their puffed cereal and lick up the caramel. Let them stabilize their plates with their hands, if necessary.

Hints

Have clean-up materials handy. Chins will become sticky.

Be sure the puffed cereal on the paper plates is at mouth level and no higher. Do not allow the children to eat with the neck tilted back or hyperextended.

Variation

Creamy peanut butter may be substituted for caramel. Place the peanut butter directly on the plate without heating or adding water.

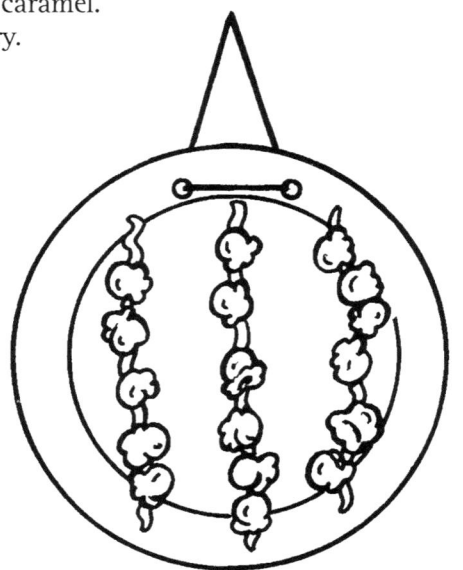

Cereal Loop Bracelets

Materials

Loop cereal

Pipe cleaners (one for each child)

Tape

Preparation

Pour the loop cereal out of the box so the children can pick it up. Give each child a pipe cleaner. Tell the children to thread cereal loops onto their pipe cleaners. When a child's pipe cleaner is 1 to 2 inches from full, twist the ends together to form a loop. Wind a 2-inch piece of tape around the twist, covering the pipe-cleaner ends.

Eating the Snack

Place the cereal bracelet on the child's wrist. Invite the child to eat the cereal off the bracelet.

Hints

Using pipe cleaners simplifies the threading task by providing stiffness. Be sure the sharp ends of the pipe cleaner are covered with tape to prevent accidents.

Colored cereal loops add interest to the activity.

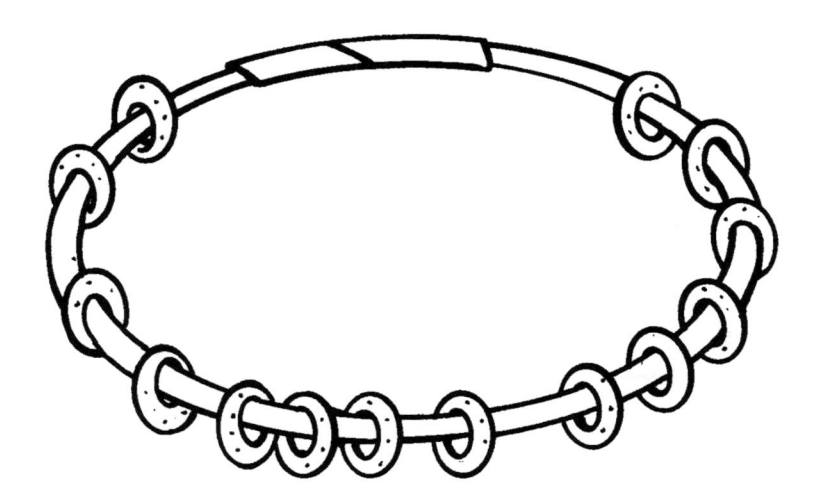

Dainty Peas

Materials

    Uncooked, thawed frozen peas (one serving for each child)

    Paper plates (one for each child)

    Flat-ended toothpicks (one for each child)

Eating the Snack

    Place the children's servings on individual plates. Give each child a toothpick. Show the children how to pierce and pick up a pea by spearing it with the toothpick. Tell the children to eat the peas one at a time. Challenge the children to remove the pea from the toothpick with their front teeth without bursting it.

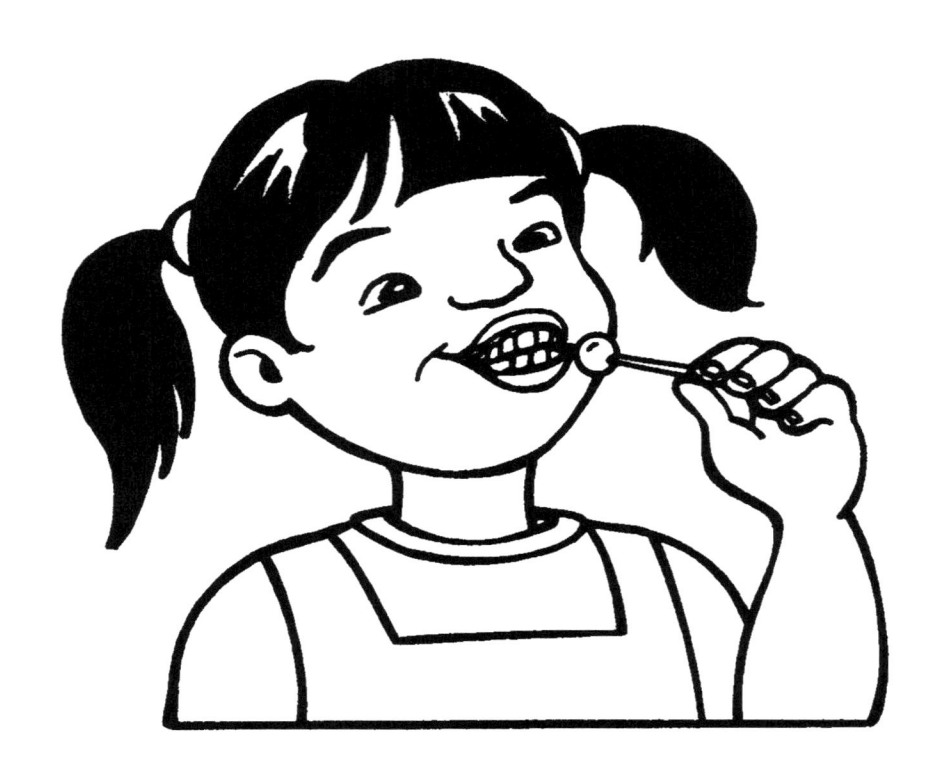

Dangling Pretzels

Materials

4-inch paper squares (one for each child)

Paper punch

A length of string (about 2 feet for each child)

Loop pretzels

Butcher paper or other protective floor covering

Preparation

Punch a hole in the center of each paper square so it can be threaded onto the string. Thread a serving of pretzels on 24 inches of string. Thread one paper square onto the string to serve as a marker. Then thread the next child's serving of pretzels on the next 24 inches of string, followed by another paper-square marker. Continue to thread the pretzels and markers, allowing 24 inches of space for each serving. Suspend the string like a clothesline at the children's chin height or below. Do not hang the pretzels higher than chin level for any child. *Do not allow any child to eat with head tilted back.* Lay the butcher paper under the suspended string.

Eating the Snack

Position one child in front of each 24-inch section of pretzels. Tell the children to eat their pretzels without using their hands. Challenge them to nibble carefully so as few pretzel pieces as possible fall onto the butcher paper on the floor. Discard fallen pretzel pieces.

Pretzels have three loops, so usually a child will manage to take several bites before breaking the loop that holds the pretzel suspended.

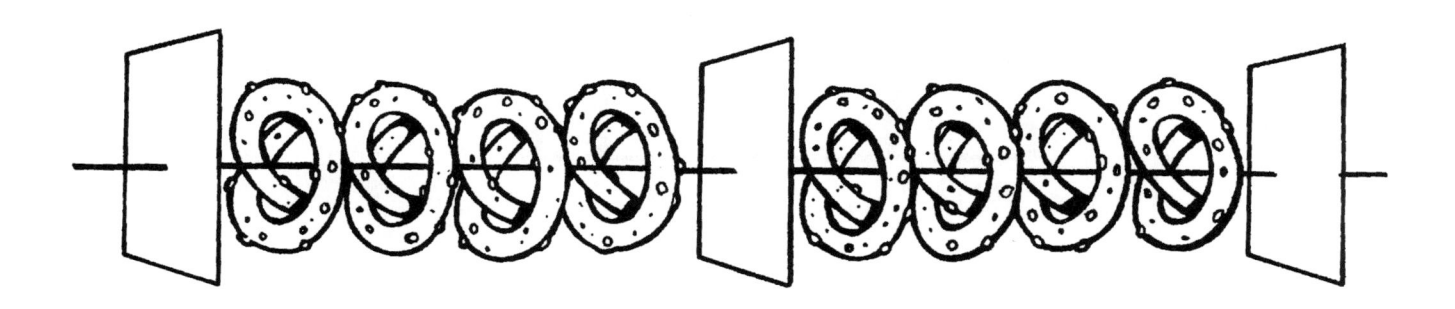

Duck's Bill Potato Chips

Materials

Stacking baked-potato chips

Eating the Snack

Place two stacking baked-potato chips wrong side together. Show the children how to place the chips in the mouth, holding them steady with the lips, not the teeth. The chips will look like a duck's bill. Invite the children to eat their duck's bills without using their hands by pulling the chips into their mouths with their lips.

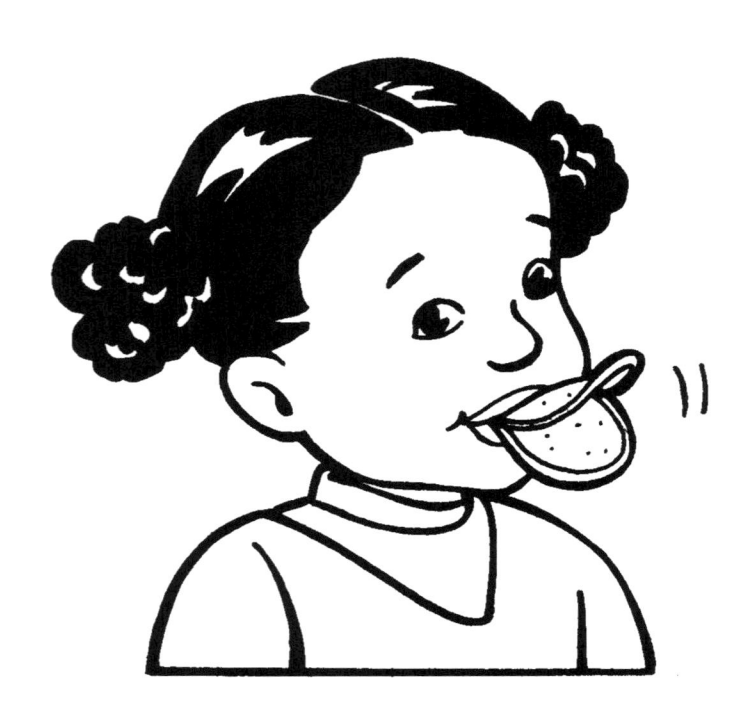

"Everybody's Done It" Spaghetti Slurp

Materials

Cooked spaghetti (one snack-sized serving for each child)

1 teaspoon vegetable oil

Bowls (one for each child)

Preparation

Cook the spaghetti and rinse it immediately in cold water. Add 1 teaspoon of vegetable oil; toss.

Eating the Snack

Set up bowls of spaghetti. Let the children slurp it up, using only their mouths.

Hint

Spaghetti may be cooked the night before and stored in plastic bags in the refrigerator.

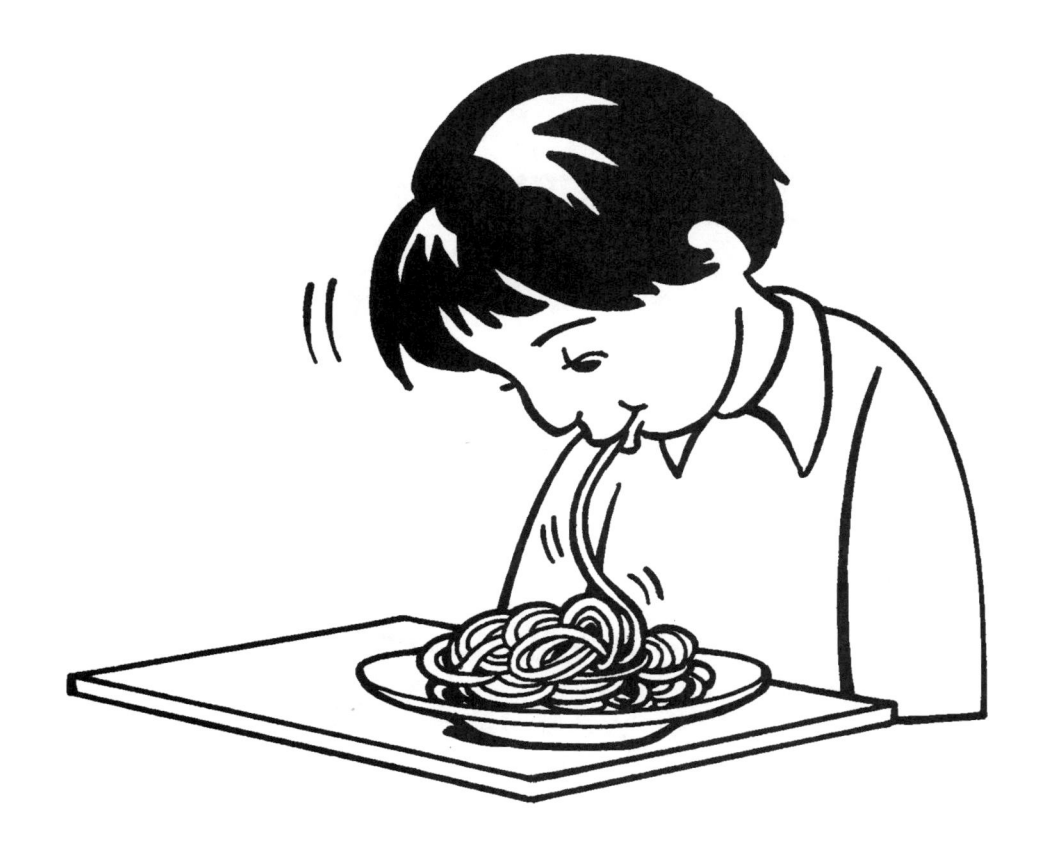

Folding Cheese

Materials

Processed or American cheese (one square for each child)

Knife

Paper plates (one for each child)

Unsweetened loop cereal (12 pieces for each child)

Preparation

Cut the square of cheese into two rectangles. Slice the rectangles across the short width, creating 12 small rectangles from each cheese square. Place these small rectangles lengthwise 1½ inches apart around the edge of a paper plate. Place the rectangles so that they hang about ¼-inch to ½-inch over the edge of the plate. When arranged, the plate will look like a sun with yellow cheese rays.

Eating the Snack

Place (or invite the children to place) one piece of unsweetened loop cereal on top of the inside end of each cheese rectangle. Tell the children to eat their cheese without using their hands. Challenge them to lift the outside end of a cheese rectangle and fold it over the cereal with their mouth before eating it.

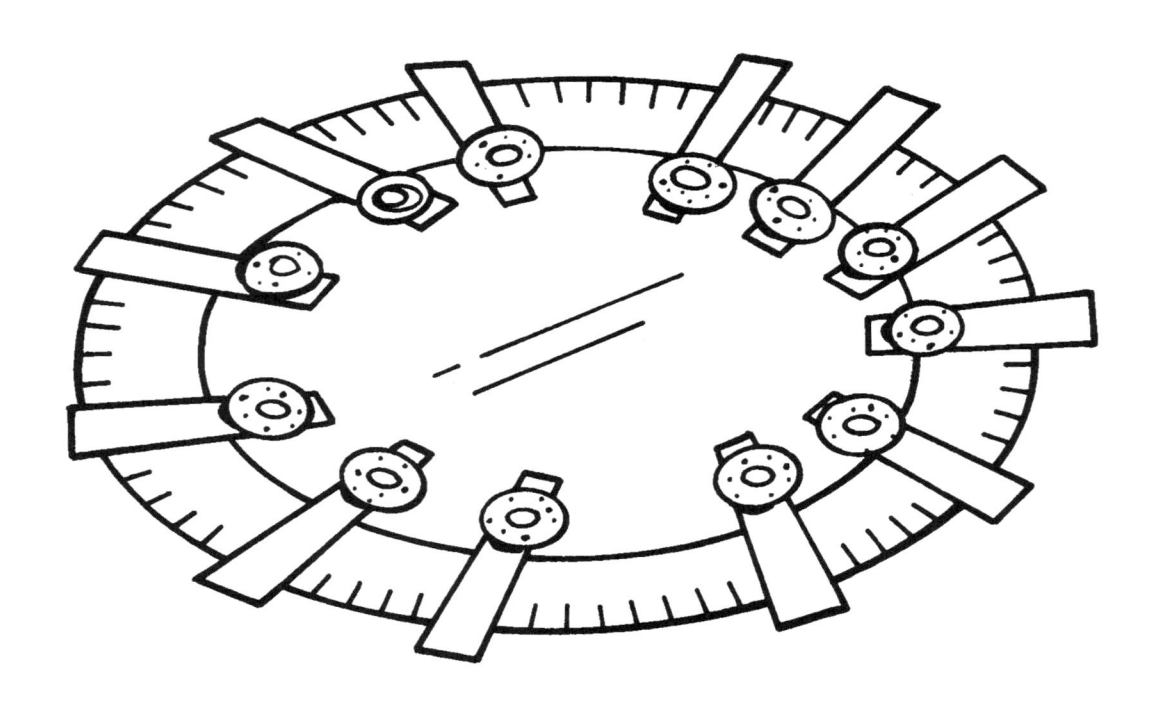

Orange-Peel Smiles

Materials

Oranges

Paring knife

Mirror

Eating the Snack

Cut the fruit into long wedges. Show the children how to bite into a wedge, hold it in their teeth, and cover it with their lips. Tell the children to look into the mirror and at each other and smile. The smile will reveal fruit peel instead of teeth.

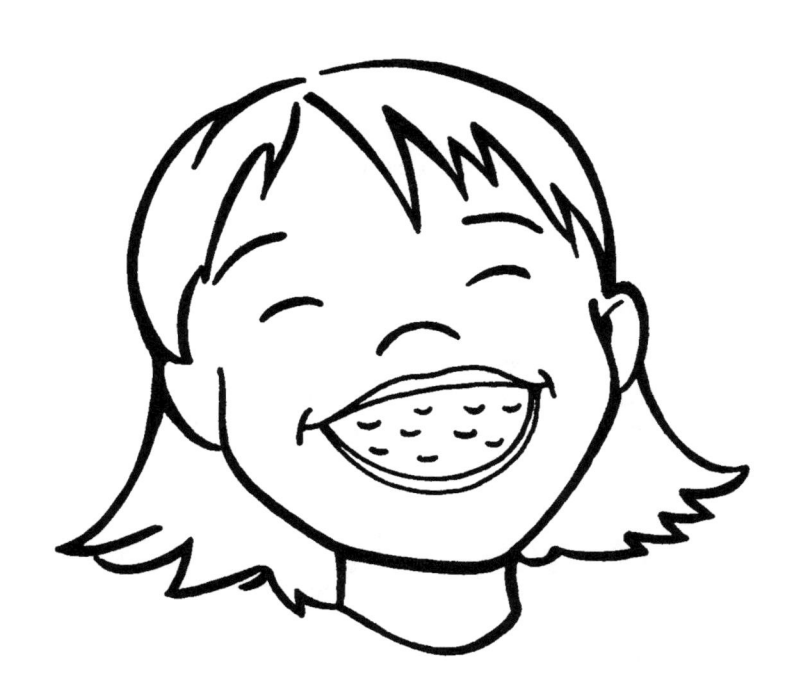

Mystery Pictures

Materials

Laminated pictures (one for each child)

Scissors

Puffed cereal

Pie plates or pans with low sides (one for each child)

Preparation

Cut a picture to fit in each pie plate. Place the pictures into the pie plates. Cover the pictures with puffed cereal.

Eating the Snack

Seat the children at the table. Give a pie plate to each child. Name an item in the picture, and tell the child to find it by eating and blowing the cereal away from that part of the picture. Direct the children to other parts of the picture. Challenge the children to be the first to eat up all the cereal over the picture.

Hints

Puffed cereal blows very easily. Placing the picture in a shallow pan will reduce cleanup.

Do not use unlaminated newsprint or ink that might become wet as the children lick their pictures.

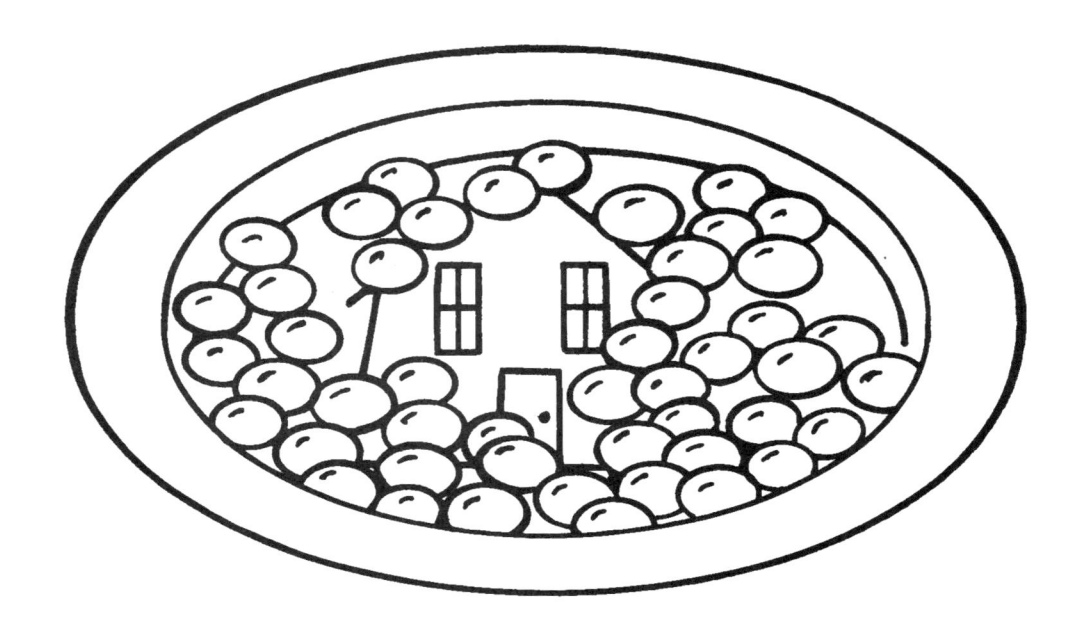

Peanut Butter Cups

Materials

Disposable cups (one for each child)

Peanut butter (one tablespoon for each child)

Preparation

Spread peanut butter around the top rim of the cup and about 1 inch down on the inside.

Eating the Snack

Give each child a peanut butter cup. Tell the children to lick up their peanut butter from inside the cup.

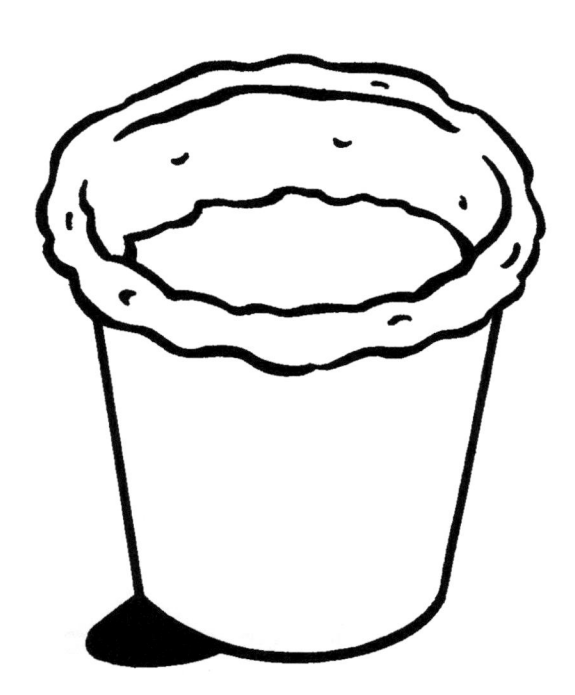

Raisin Anteater Trail

Materials

Sheet of clean butcher paper

Raisins

Eating the Snack

Lay the sheet of clean butcher paper on the floor. Assemble the children on the floor on one side of the butcher paper. Drop a trail of raisins across the butcher paper for each child. Tell the children, "You are anteaters, and the raisins are ants. Anteaters lick up ants with their tongues." Have the children crawl across the paper while they eat their trail of ants, using only their mouths.

Variations

To avoid the chewy consistency of raisins, use cocoa-flavored cereal pieces.

For a sweet treat, use chocolate chips as ants.

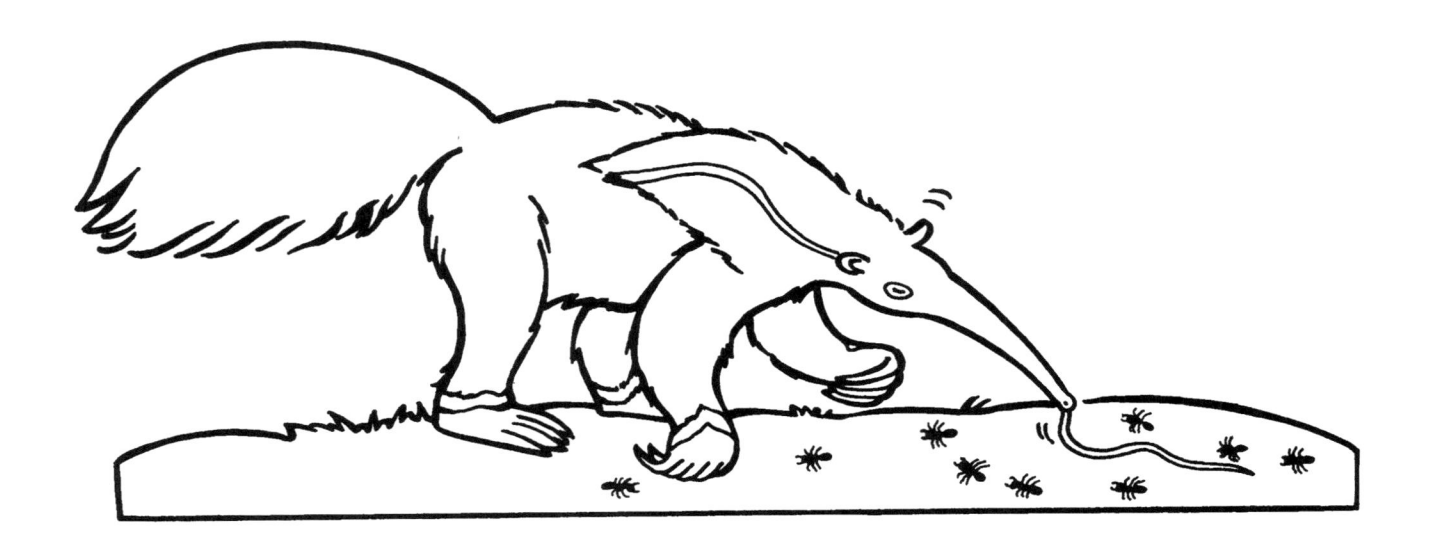

Squeeze-Cheese Trails

Materials

Finger-painting paper (one sheet for each child)

Tape

Soft cheese in a squeeze dispenser

Eating the Snack

Seat the children at the table. Tape a sheet of finger-painting paper in front of each child. Dispense the cheese to the paper and draw a pattern of squiggly lines or a face. Tell the children to lick up the cheese.

It is important to choose a slick paper that is not water-absorbent. Avoid colored paper or paper with dyes that might become part of the cheese. Match the cheese drawings to the topic of the week.

Variation

Dispatch a monster by face part—eyes first, then the nose, finally the mouth.

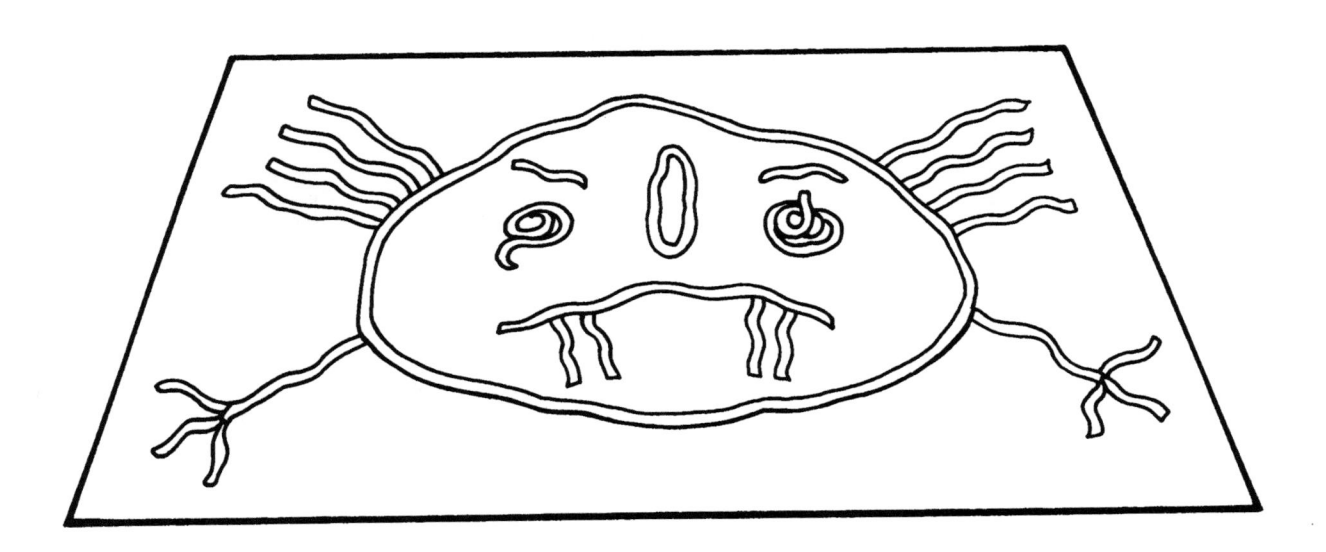

Stacking Marshmallow Blocks

Materials

Marshmallows (three for each child)

Clean sheets of paper (one for each child)

Tape

Eating the Snack

Seat the children at the table. Tape a clean sheet of paper in front of each child. Give each child three marshmallows. Tell the children to build a tower with their marshmallows. Show the children how to pick up the marshmallows with their mouths and stack one on top of another. When the towers are made, tell the children to eat them down, one marshmallow at a time.

Hint

Marshmallows are slanted on the top, so this task is not as easy as it seems. To assist the children, press a slanted marshmallow, using the flat of your hand. Often it will pop back up with a straighter top.

Variation

For a higher challenge, use miniature marshmallows. These are more difficult not only because of their size, but because you cannot see them as you stack them with your mouth.

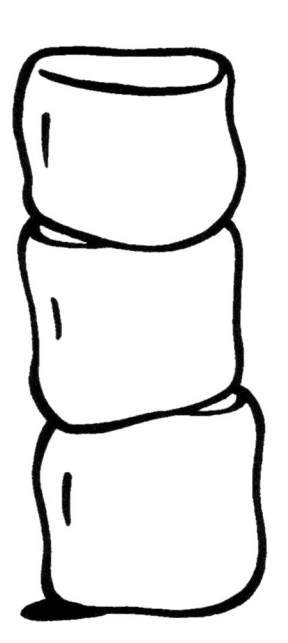

Sweet Goat Nibbles

Materials

Finger-painting paper (one sheet for each child)

Tape

Pastel cake decorations or jimmies (one tablespoon for each child)

Eating the Snack

Seat the children at the table. Tape a sheet of finger-painting paper in front of each child. Scatter a tablespoon of cake decorations on the paper for each child. Tell the children, "You are goats, and this is your pasture." Have the children eat the "nibbles" without using their hands. Let them make goat noises.

The children may choose to lick up the decorations. Encourage them to nibble them with their lips like goats.

Variation

For a healthful substitute, use shredded lettuce and carrots.

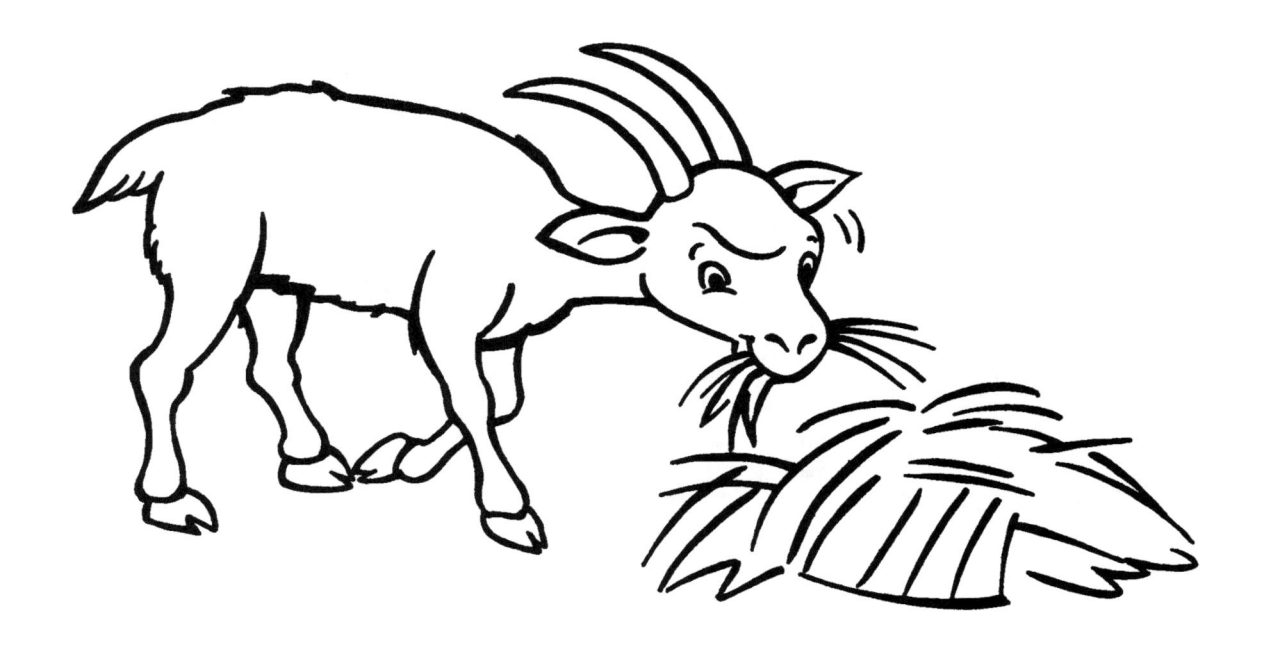

Dog-Bowl Races

Materials

Chalk

Pudding

Serving spoon

Shallow bowls (one for each child)

Eating the Snack

Mark START and FINISH lines on the floor about 10 feet apart. Have the children line up on the floor in all-fours position. Put a dollop of pudding in a bowl for each child.

Place the bowls on the floor, one in front of each child. Tell the children to crawl forward and use only their mouths to move their bowls across the FINISH line while simultaneously licking up the pudding.

Hints

Adjust the length of the race to the amount of pudding. Make the FINISH line a turn-around point to challenge the children further in organizing their movements. End the trail against a wall; this will stabilize the bowls so the children can finish their pudding.

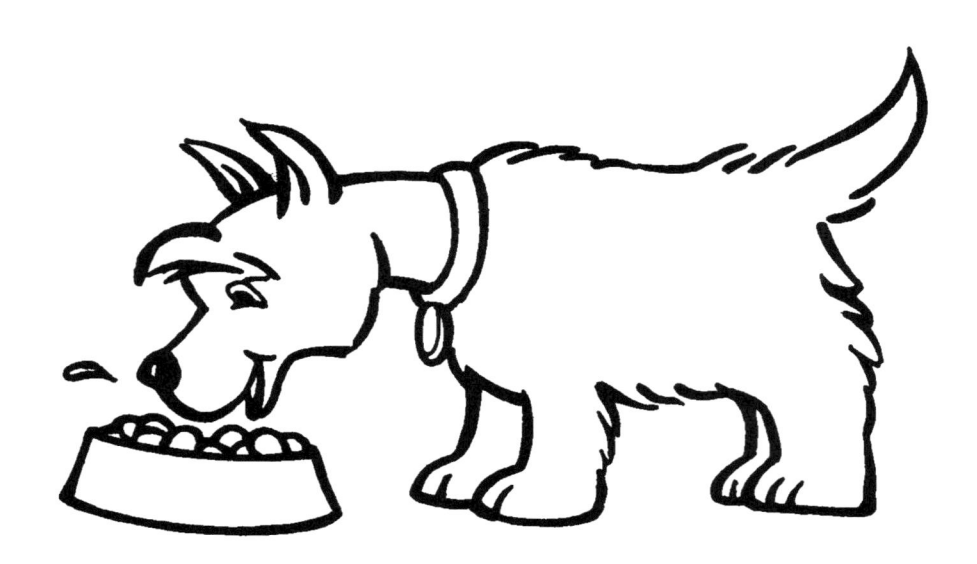

Whipped Cream All Over

Materials

Whipped cream in a can dispenser

Paper towels, soap, and water for cleanup

Eating the Snack

Have the children wash their hands. Seat the children at a table. Tell them to hold their hands up and spread their fingers. Dispense a blob of whipped cream on each of the children's fingertips. Place a blob of cream at the corners of each child's mouth by dispensing the cream first to your fingertip and then to the child. Wash your hands after touching each child's mouth. Tell the children to eat!

Encourage the children to try to lick the whipped cream off the edges of their mouths first. This will challenge them to use their tongues and not their fingers to do this.

Hint

This is a sticky activity! Warm soap and water will be needed for cleanup.

Variation

Vary the activity by singing the song, "Where Is Thumbkin?" Have the children lick the whipped cream off the fingers in sequence.

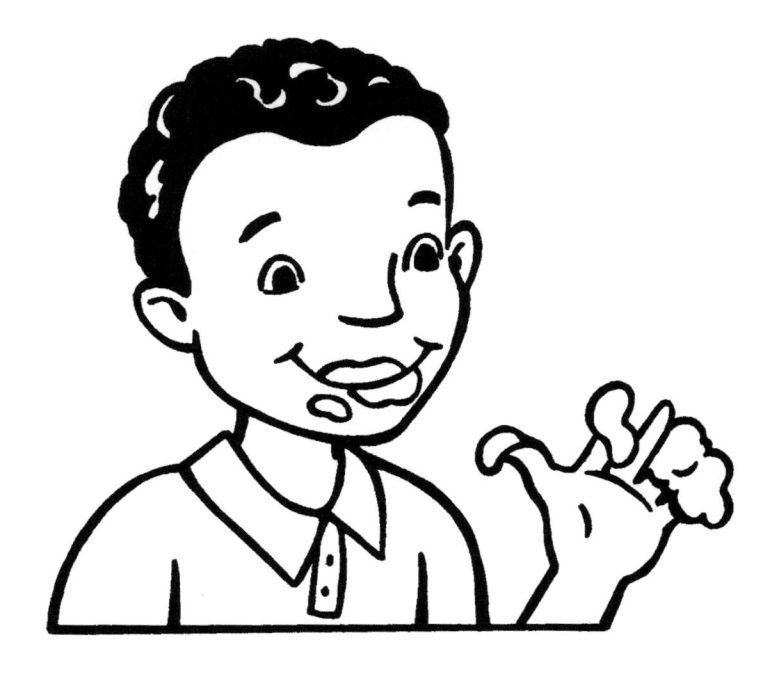

Alliteration Songs

About the Alliteration Songs

Each alliteration song is based on a consonant sound. In each song, the consonant sound is combined with several vowel phonemes. To increase the children's interest, each alliteration song is matched with a game or an action.

Alliteration songs work best in a group setting. Children often are motivated to participate and sing with their peers. Alliteration songs provide the best practice when they are sung frequently. Familiarity with the songs improves the rate of participation. Include the songs as part of other daily group activities, and use them during the children's regular singing time.

In many of the alliteration songs, an individual child is chosen to perform a special action. The desire to perform can be motivating to some children and frightening to others. Do not force children to participate as a leader. Children who do not join the group readily often come forward after watching others play the game many times. Familiarity overcomes reluctance.

Alliteration songs provide opportunities to connect oral motor movements with forming words. Speech movement can be learned only within the context of speech. The songs provide practice in making consonant sounds in various combinations.

Alliteration Warm-Ups

Magic Fingers

Hold up your fingers and wiggle them. Say to the children, "Magic fingers, rub my forehead." Lead the children in massaging their foreheads. Then have the magic fingers rub other parts of the face, eyebrows, ears, cheeks, jaw, and nose. Massage the mouth by twiddling the lips ("Brrr-blll-brrr-blll!").

Motor Boat Song

Sing the song, "Row, Row, Row Your Boat" five times, substituting the words "Putt, putt, putt your boat" the first time. Repeat the song, dropping the words on the first line and replacing them with raspberry noises ("Brrr"). The next time, drop the words on the first and second line; and so on, until the entire song is a series of raspberries.

Bee Bobble Bibble Bobble Boo!

Material

A bean bag

Playing the Game

Seat the children in a circle. Call one child to the center of the circle. Place a bean bag on the child's head. All the children sing the first three lines of the song. After the line, "I asked him (her) a question, and this is what she (he) said," the child in the center replies. "Bee bobble bibble bobble boo." If a child is reluctant to sing alone, encourage the child to sing this line quietly in your ear. With familiarity, the children will become more relaxed with singing this line in front of an audience. After singing the reply, the child in the center of the group skips around the circle while the entire group sings the chorus. At the end of the song, the another child is chosen and the game is played again.

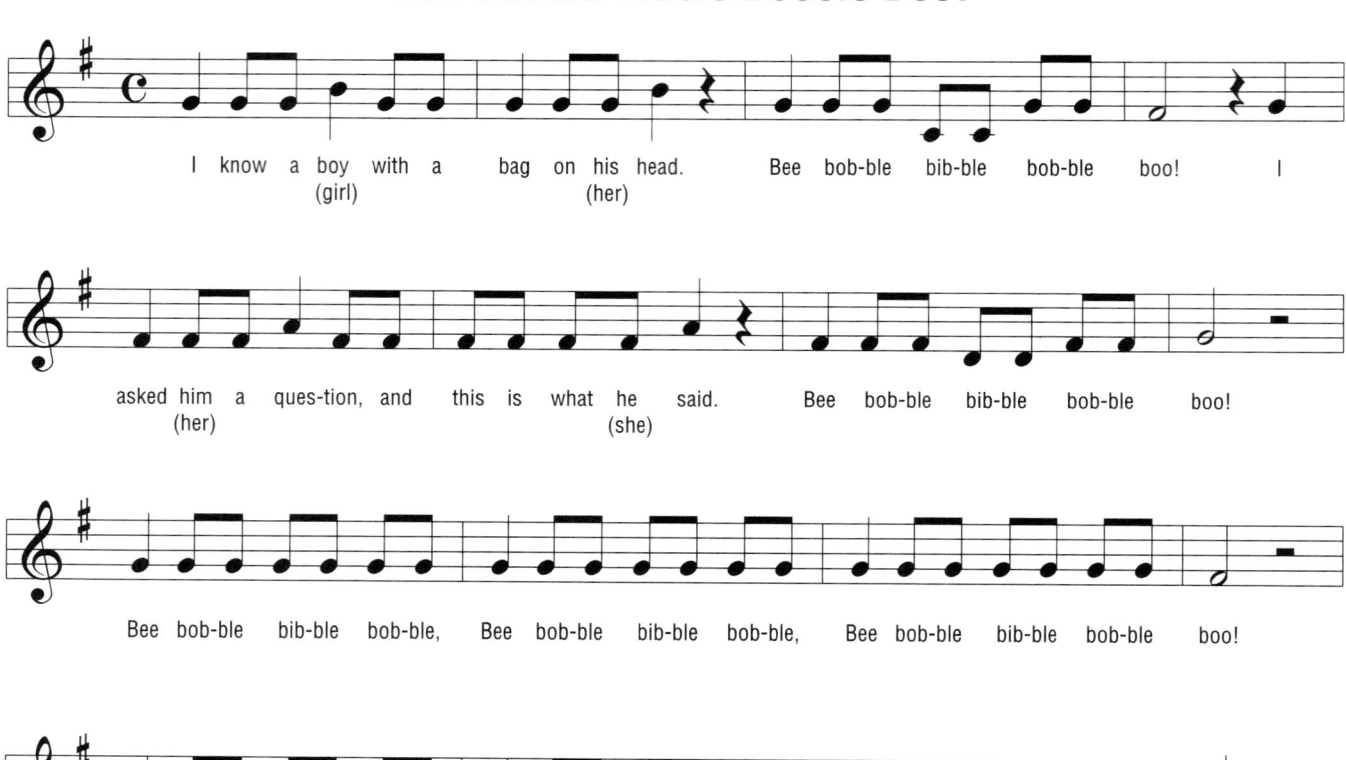

Bee Bobble Bibble Bobble Boo!

I know a boy with a bag on his head. Bee bob-ble bib-ble bob-ble boo! I
(girl)   (her)

asked him a ques-tion, and this is what he said. Bee bob-ble bib-ble bob-ble boo!
(her)   (she)

Bee bob-ble bib-ble bob-ble, Bee bob-ble bib-ble bob-ble, Bee bob-ble bib-ble bob-ble boo!

Bee bob-ble bib-ble bob-ble, Bee bob-ble bib-ble bob-ble, Bee bob-ble bib-ble bob-ble boo!

Chewy–Chewy Chaw

Material

A bean bag or small pillow

Playing the Game

Seat the children in a circle facing each other. One child has the "chaw" (the bean bag or pillow). As the children sing the song, they clap their hands on the word *chaw*. At the end of the song, the children shout the phrase, "Chuck it!" The child with the pillow tosses it to another child, and the song is repeated.

Chewy–Chewy Chaw

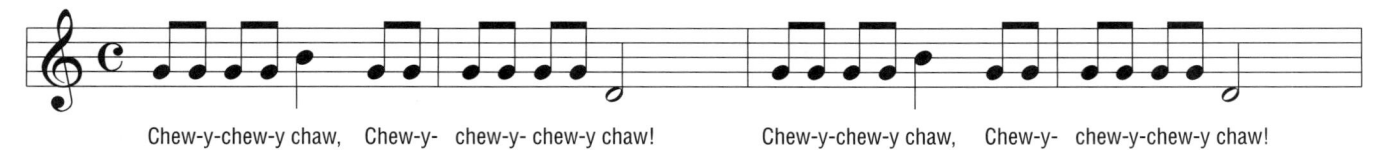

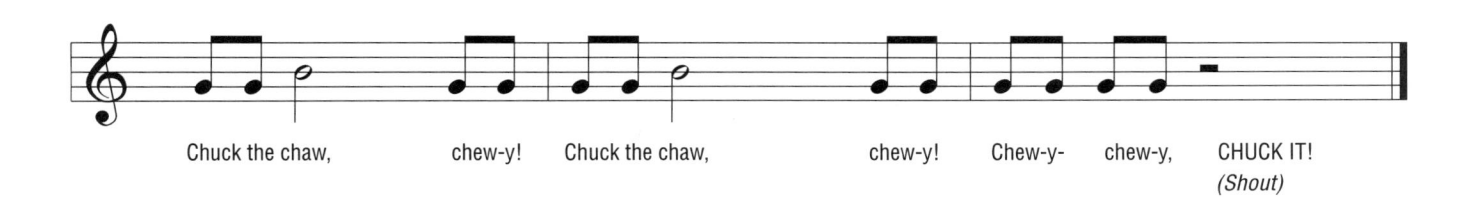

Chew-y-chew-y chaw, Chew-y- chew-y- chew-y chaw! Chew-y-chew-y chaw, Chew-y- chew-y-chew-y chaw!

Chuck the chaw, chew-y! Chuck the chaw, chew-y! Chew-y- chew-y, CHUCK IT!
(Shout)

Derry-Down-Nitty

Singing the Song

Sing the first six lines in this song, and have the children initiate the chorus by shouting "Again!" The entire group then sings the chorus. At the end of the chorus, the children shout "Again!" once more, and all sing the chorus. Repeat the chorus as long as interest continues.

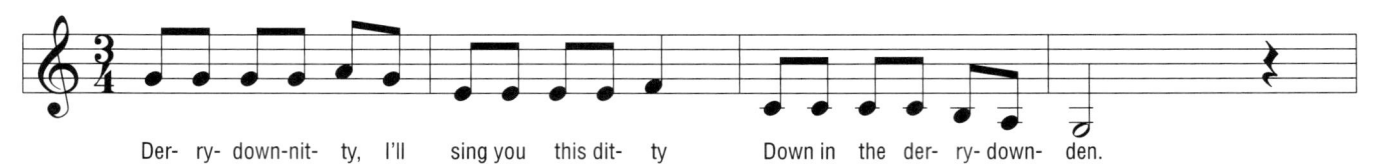

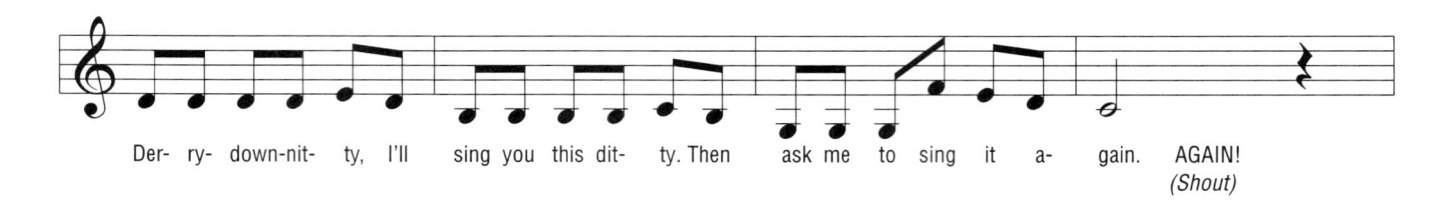

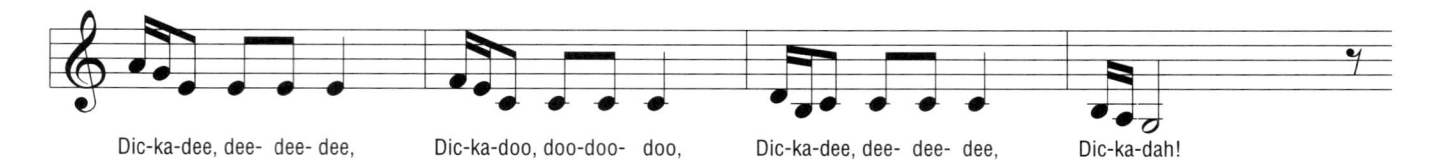

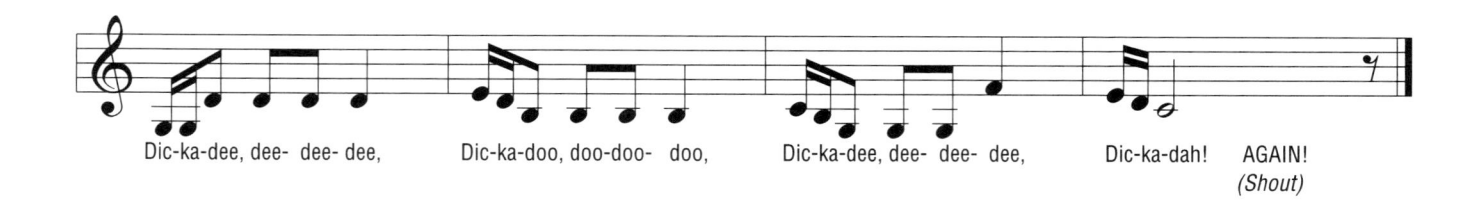

Derry-Down-Nitty

Der-ry-down-nit-ty, I'll sing you this dit-ty Down in the der-ry-down-den.

Der-ry-down-nit-ty, I'll sing you this dit-ty. Then ask me to sing it a-gain. AGAIN! (Shout)

Dic-ka-dee, dee-dee-dee, Dic-ka-doo, doo-doo-doo, Dic-ka-dee, dee-dee-dee, Dic-ka-dah!

Dic-ka-dee, dee-dee-dee, Dic-ka-doo, doo-doo-doo, Dic-ka-dee, dee-dee-dee, Dic-ka-dah! AGAIN! (Shout)

Fingle, Flyger, Feather Stuff

Playing the Game

Repeat the verse three times with accompanying hand actions. The action on the first three lines changes with each repetition. The first time the song is sung, the group claps one hand on one leg throughout. The second time, the group alternates claps, one hand on one leg, then the other hand on the other leg, throughout the first three lines. The third time, the two leg claps are followed by a hand clap throughout the first three lines. For all three times, both hands are raised to the ears and waved back while singing, "Flip it up" and the arms are rolled while singing "Flip it over." For "Ffffff! Ffffff! Ffffff!" the children place their index fingers under their noses ready to sneeze for the "Achoo!"

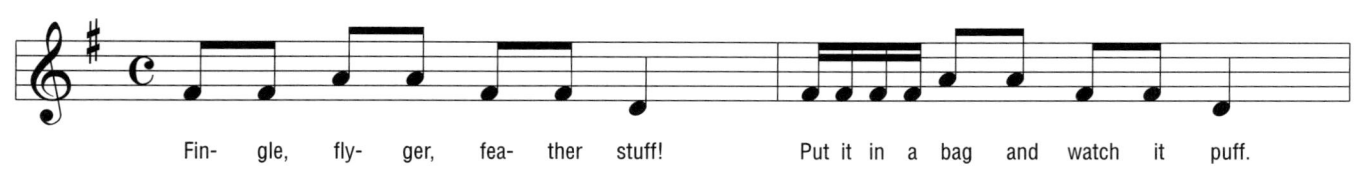

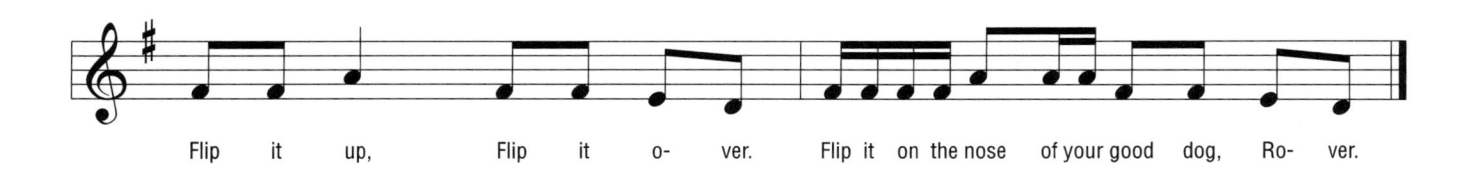

Fingle, Flyger, Feather Stuff

Fin- gle, fly- ger, fea- ther stuff! Put it in a bag and watch it puff.

Flip it up, Flip it o- ver. Flip it on the nose of your good dog, Ro- ver.

(Voiced) **Ffffff! Ffffff! Ffffff! ACHOO!**

Goop

Singing the Song

This song is sung as a round, in which half of the singing group sings the verse while the other half simultaneously sings the chorus. Children will need some familiarity with the song before they attempt this harmonizing split. To facilitate the activity, have two leaders—one for each part.

Goop

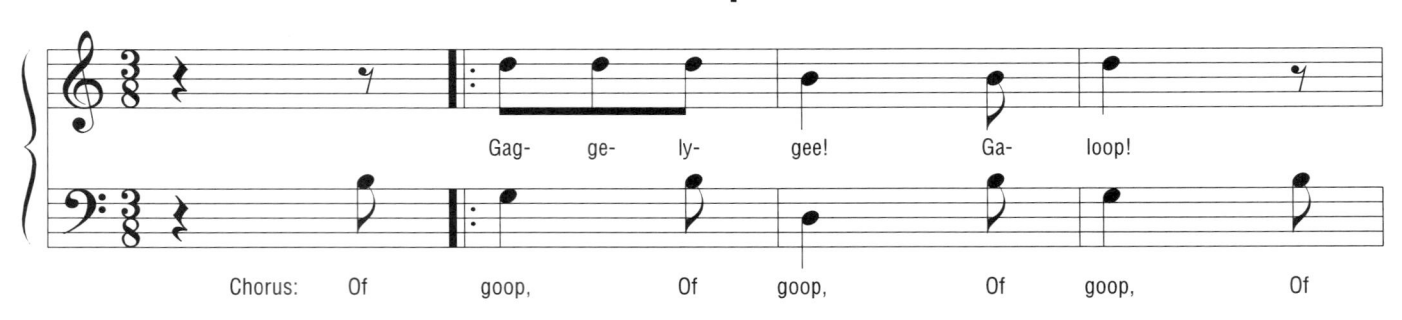

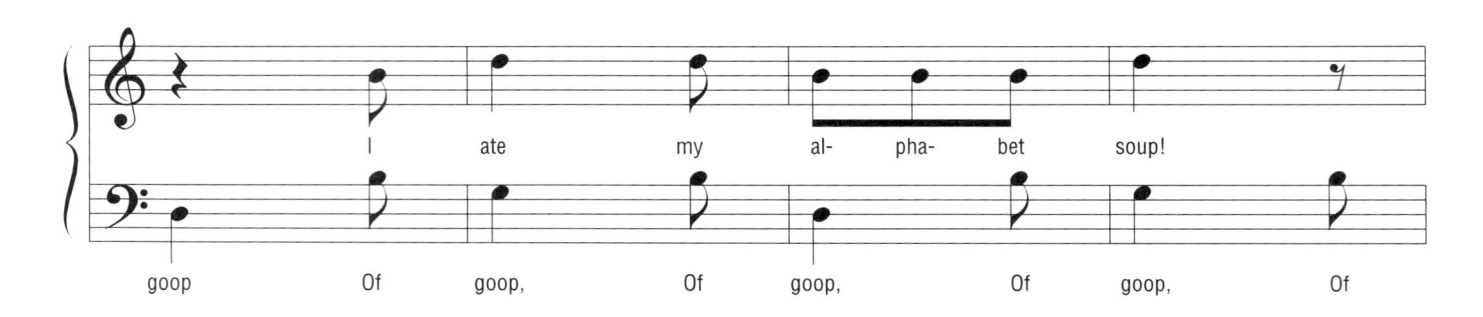

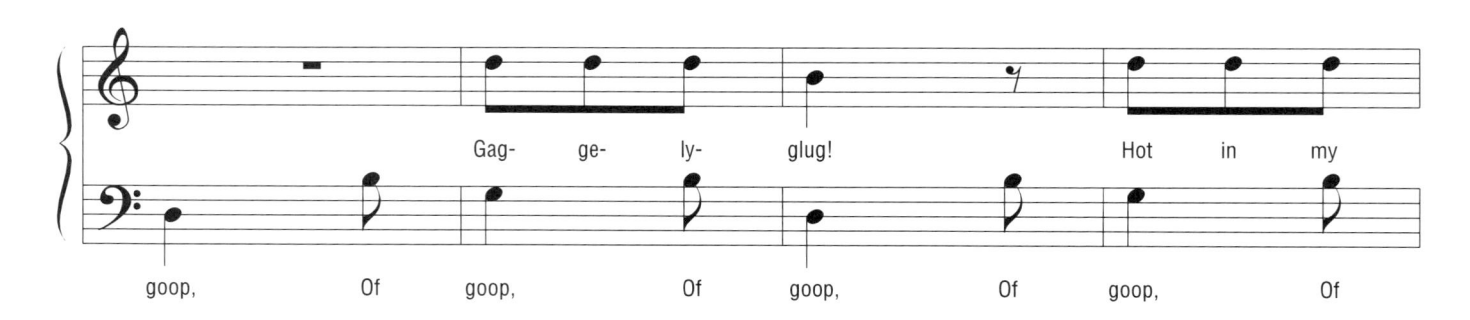

Chorus: Of goop, Of goop, Of goop, Of goop Of goop, Of goop, Of goop, Of goop, Of goop, Of goop, Of goop, Of

Gag-ge-ly-gee! Ga-loop! I ate my al-pha-bet soup! Gag-ge-ly-glug! Hot in my

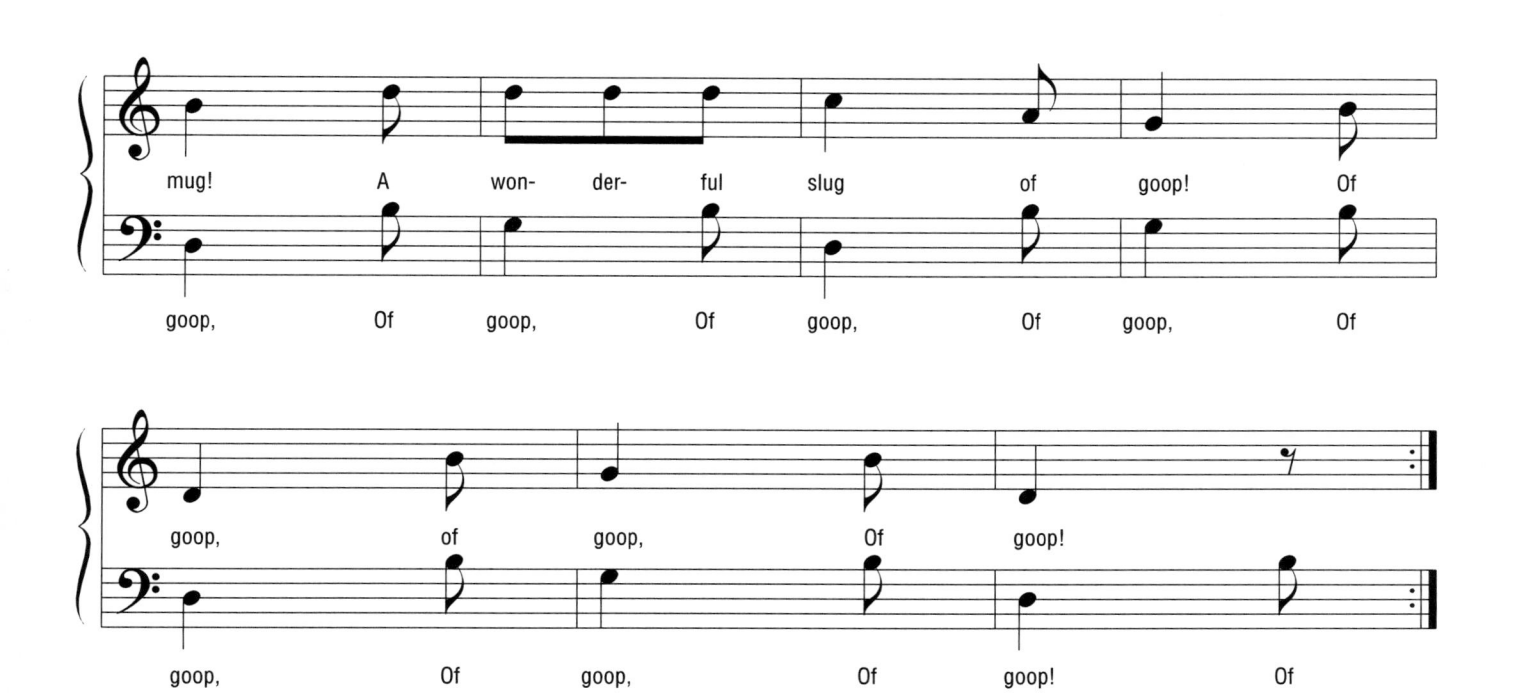

mug! A won- der- ful slug of goop! Of
goop, Of goop, Of goop, Of goop, Of

goop, of goop, Of goop! Of
goop, Of goop, Of goop! Of

My Old Mule, Hugh

Playing the Game

Seat the children in a circle. Call one child to stand in the center of the circle. As the group sings, "He walks high," the child in the center stretches up on tiptoes. When the children sing, "He walks low," the child in the center crouches down. As the group sings, "He walks to, and he walks fro," the child in the center paces back and forth. As the children sing, "Hey-hee, hi-ho," the selected child spins in the middle of the circle. On "Hugh," the child stops the spin and points to another child in the circle. The first child sits down and the newly selected child takes the center position. The new child is asked to choose a different animal, and the new animal name (lion, turtle, dog, . . .) is sung in place of the word *mule*. The game continues as long as interest continues.

My Old Mule, Hugh

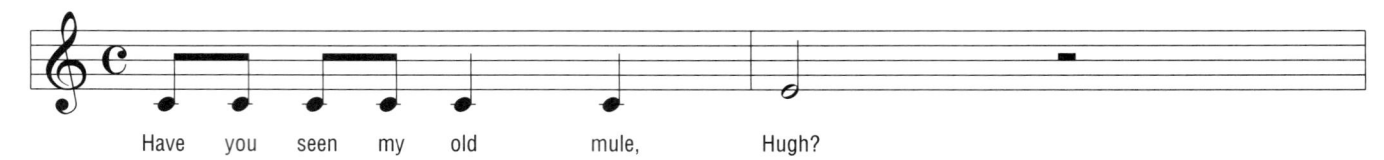

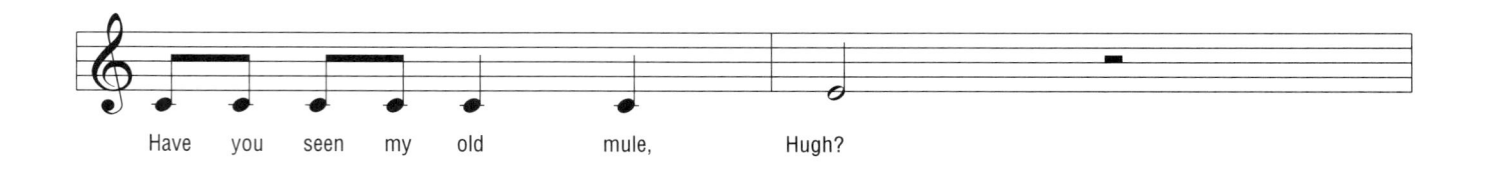

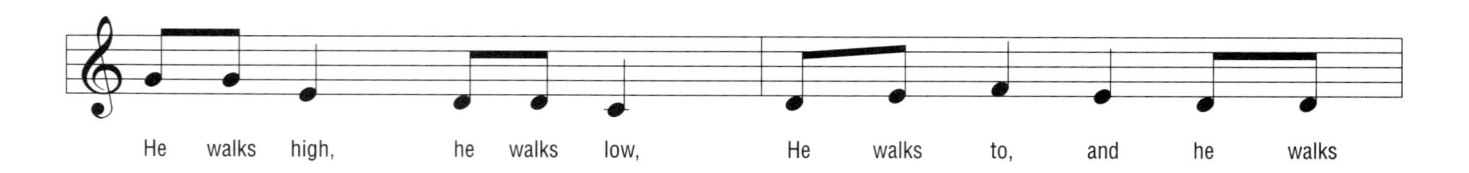

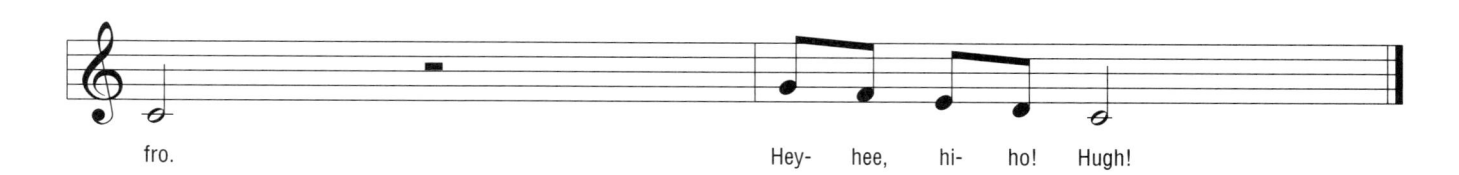

Have you seen my old mule, Hugh?

Have you seen my old mule, Hugh?

He walks high, he walks low, He walks to, and he walks fro.

Hey-hee, hi-ho! Hugh!

Jolly Jiggles

Playing the Game

Seat the children in a circle. As they sing this song, the children jiggle their bodies and bounce to the rhythm. On the word *jolt,* they give an extra bounce to their jiggle. On the last line, this extra bounce turns into a topple as they finish the song by falling over.

Jolly Jiggles

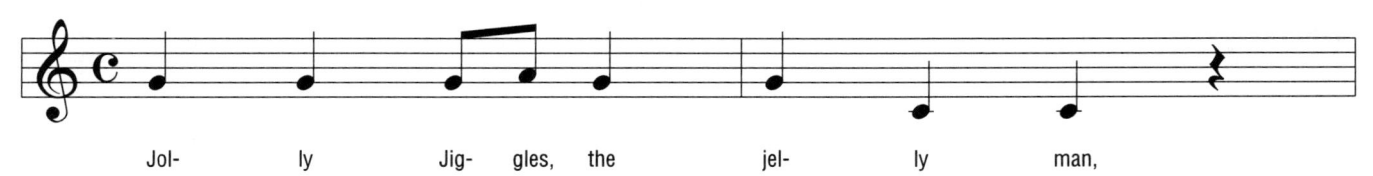

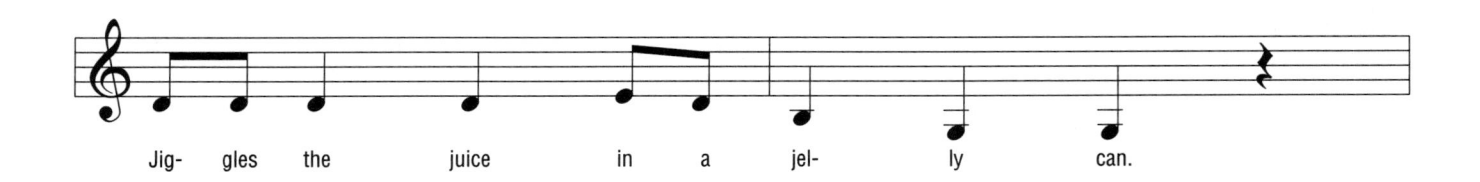

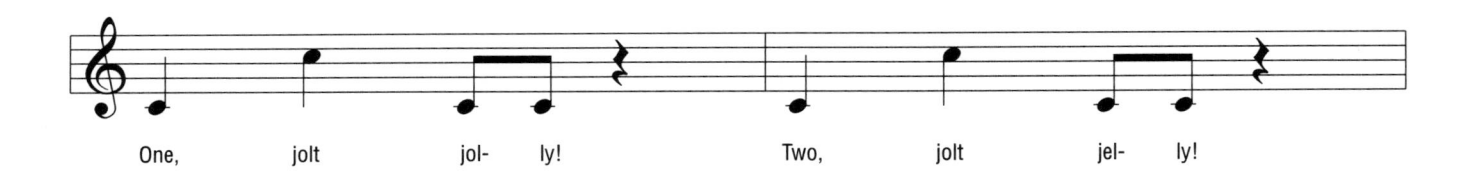

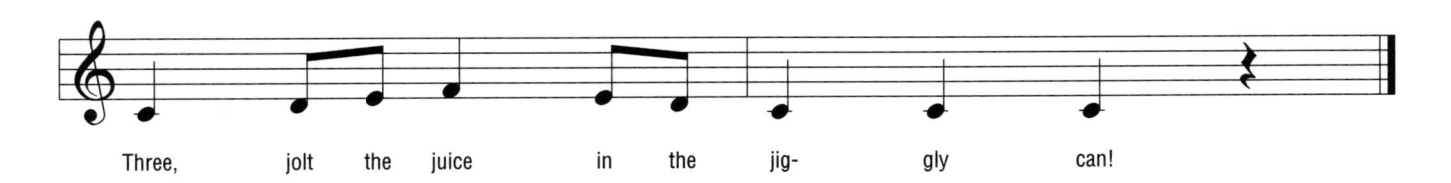

Jol- ly Jig- gles, the jel- ly man,

Jig- gles the juice in a jel- ly can.

One, jolt jol- ly! Two, jolt jel- ly!

Three, jolt the juice in the jig- gly can!

Kuh-Kuh-Kuh-Roo!

Playing the Game

One child stands in front of the others through the opening verse. At the chorus, the standing child scratches the ground with the feet and flaps the arms like wings on a chicken. Select another child, and repeat the song.

Kuh-Kuh-Kuh-Roo!

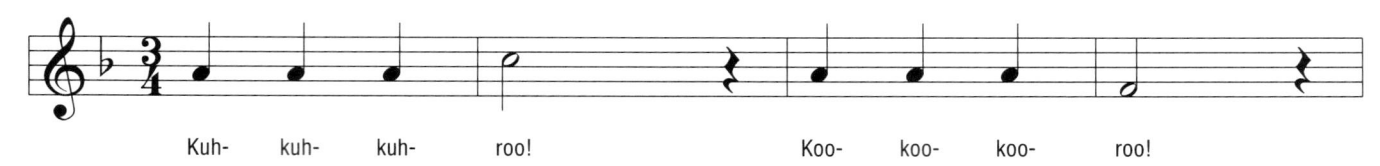

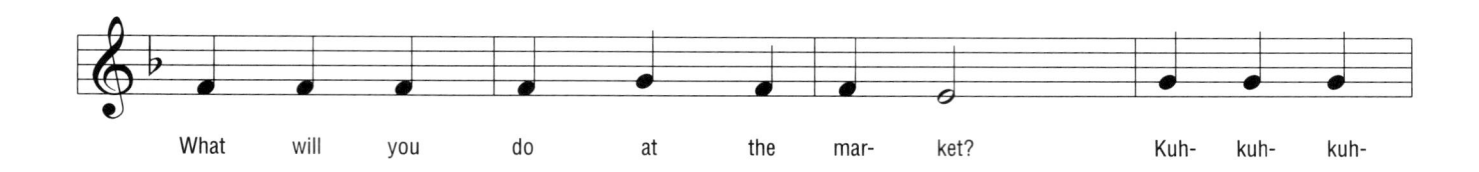

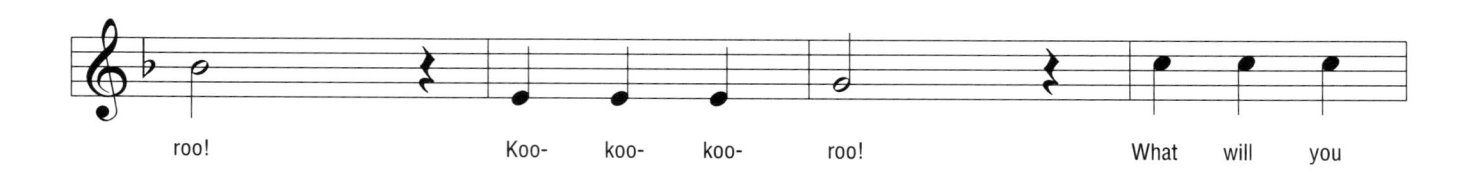

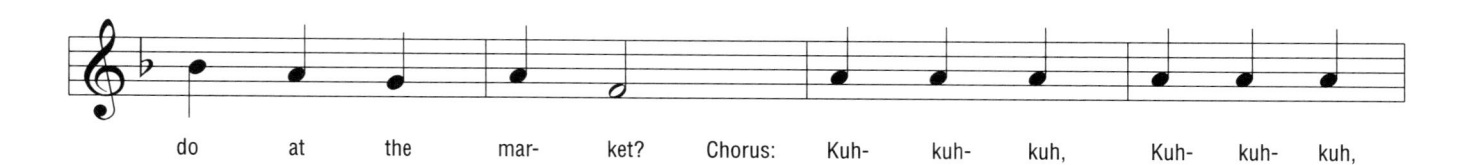

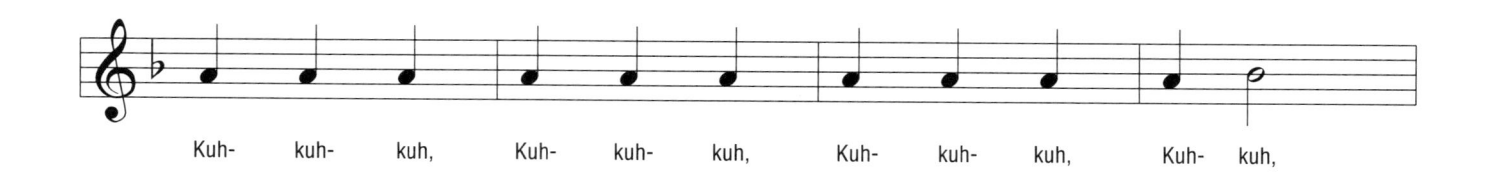

Kuh- kuh- kuh- roo! Koo- koo- koo- roo!
What will you do at the mar- ket? Kuh- kuh- kuh-
roo! Koo- koo- koo- roo! What will you
do at the mar- ket? Chorus: Kuh- kuh- kuh, Kuh- kuh- kuh,
Kuh- kuh- kuh, Kuh- kuh- kuh, Kuh- kuh- kuh, Kuh- kuh,

Kay- daa- ket! Kuh- kuh- kuh, Kuh- kuh- kuh, Kuh- kuh- kuh,

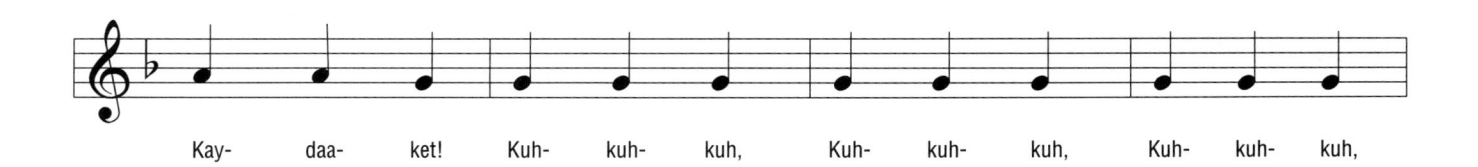

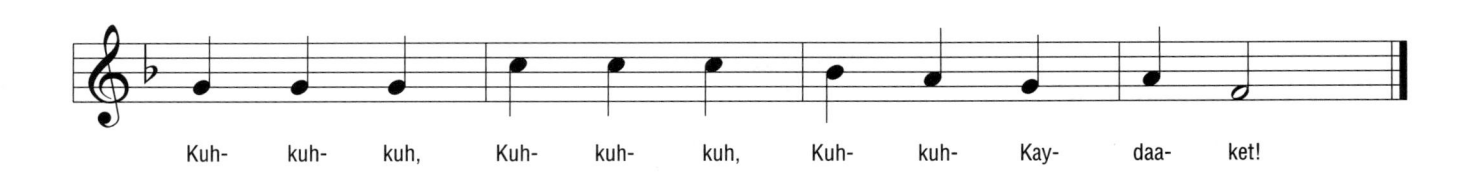

Kuh- kuh- kuh, Kuh- kuh- kuh, Kuh- kuh- Kay- daa- ket!

Lulla-Baby

Singing the Song

This song is sung responsively. Have the children form two groups. Seat the groups in lines across from one another. Both groups sing the "Lulla-baby" lines together. For the chorus, one group sings, "La-la" and the other group responds, "La-la." Repeat; then both groups sing "La-la-la-la-la" together. They sing the chorus twice.

Another option is to sing responsively between the group and one child. If the child is reluctant to sing alone, encourage the child to sing this line quietly in your ear. With familiarity, the children will become more relaxed with singing responsively for an audience.

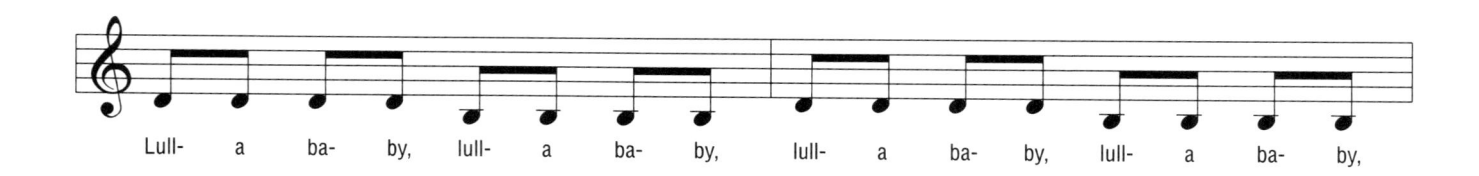

Lulla-Baby

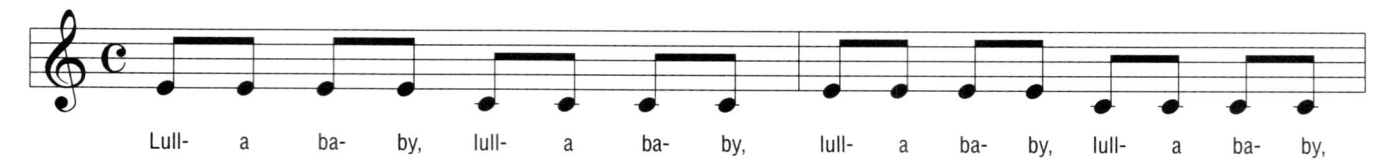

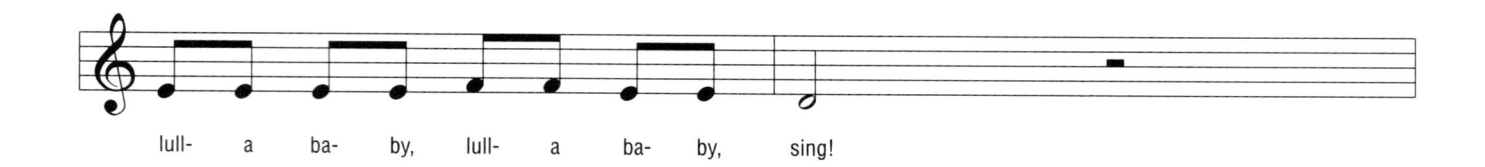

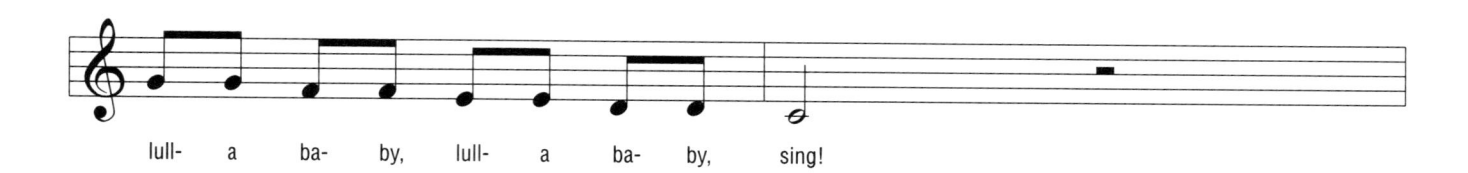

Lull- a ba- by, lull- a ba- by, lull- a ba- by, lull- a ba- by,

lull- a ba- by, lull- a ba- by, sing!

Lull- a ba- by, lull- a ba- by, lull- a ba- by, lull- a ba- by,

lull- a ba- by, lull- a ba- by, sing!

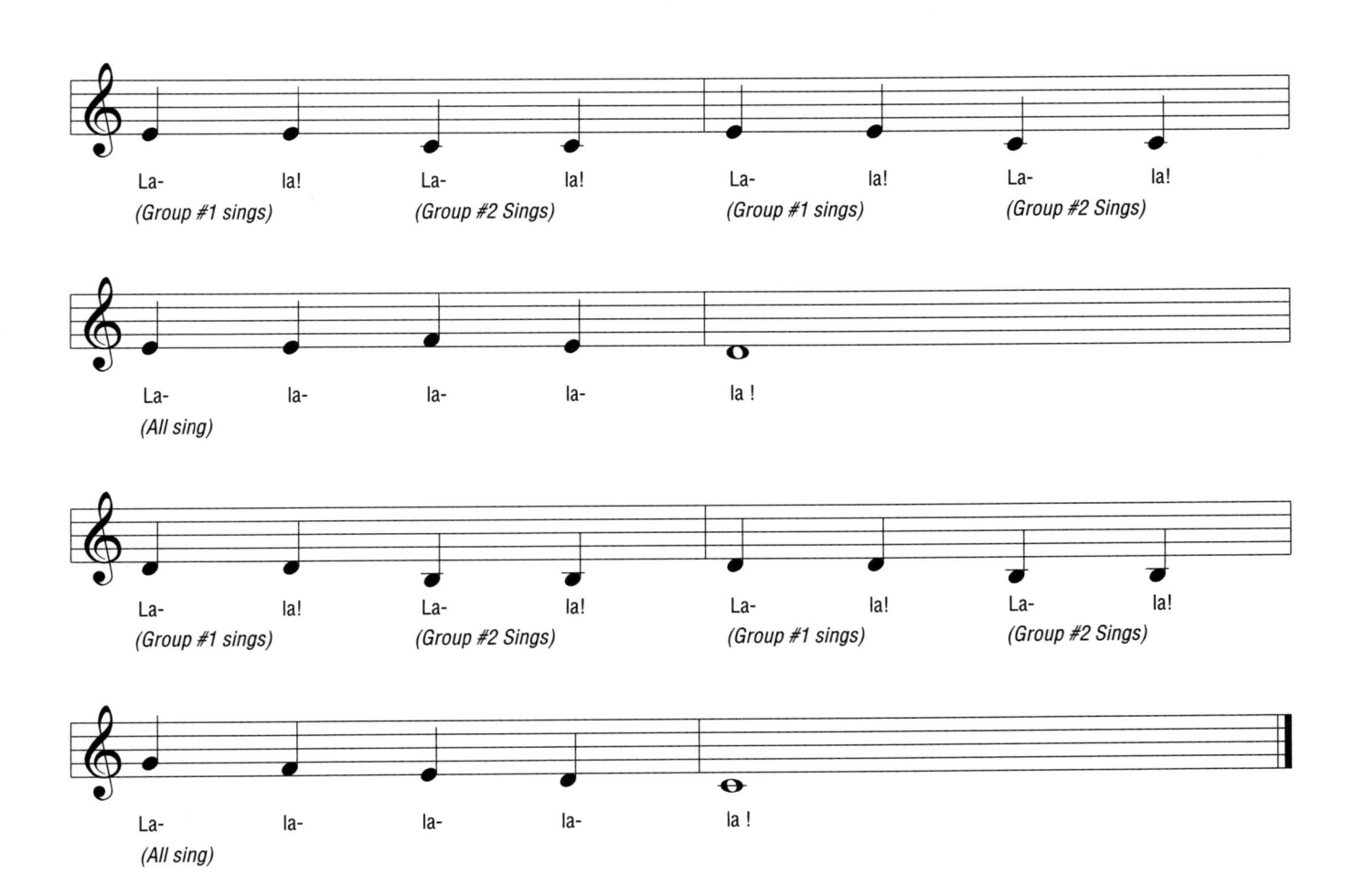

La- la! La- la! La- la! La- la!
(Group #1 sings) *(Group #2 Sings)* *(Group #1 sings)* *(Group #2 Sings)*

La- la- la- la- la !
(All sing)

La- la! La- la! La- la! La- la!
(Group #1 sings) *(Group #2 Sings)* *(Group #1 sings)* *(Group #2 Sings)*

La- la- la- la- la !
(All sing)

Mounds of Mushy Fruit

Playing the Game

Seat the children in a circle. Call one child to stand in the center of the circle. All sing the verse together as the child in the center skips around the inside of the circle. On the chorus, the child in the center rocks back and forth as all sing "Mmmm" and stomps on the ground for "Mounds of mushy fruit." At the end of the chorus, the child in the center pretends to slip on the mushy fruit and falls to the ground. The child points to another child, and the song is repeated.

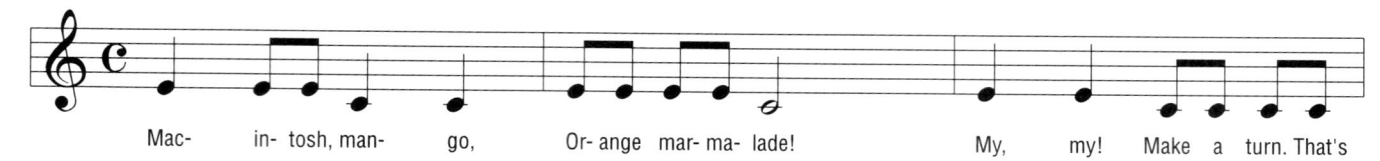

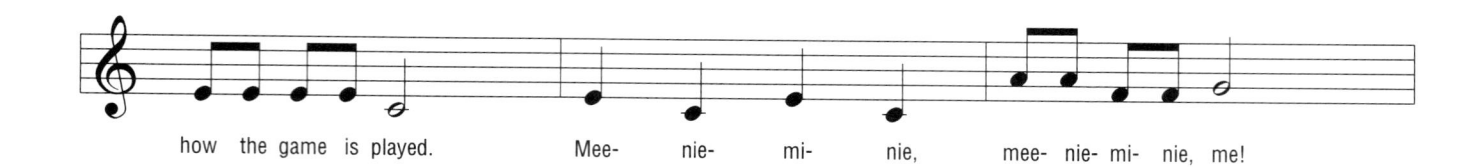

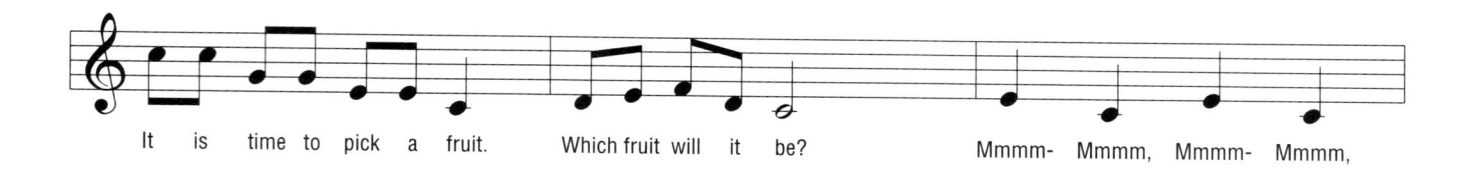

Mounds of Mushy Fruit

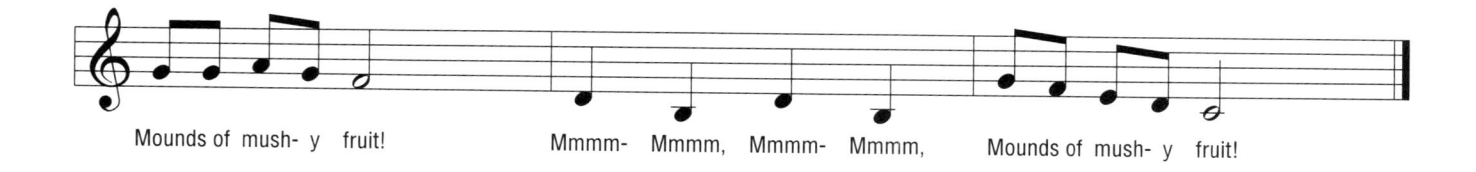

Mac-in-tosh, man-go, Or-ange mar-ma-lade! My, my! Make a turn. That's how the game is played. Mee-nie-mi-nie, mee-nie-mi-nie, me! It is time to pick a fruit. Which fruit will it be? Mmmm-Mmmm, Mmmm-Mmmm, Mounds of mush-y fruit! Mmmm-Mmmm, Mmmm-Mmmm, Mounds of mush-y fruit!

Ninny-Nanny-Noo!

Playing the Game

Seat the children in a circle. Call one child to walk around the outside of the circle as the verse is sung. On the last word, "NOO," the walking child taps a sitting child. The sitting child rises and chases the walking child around the outside of the circle. As the two children run, the group chants, "Ninny-nanny, ninny-nanny," until the first child reaches the empty place in the circle and sits down. At that moment, the chant ends with "NOO!" The child left standing now walks the outside of the circle as the game is repeated.

Ninny-Nanny-Noo!

Nin-ny-nan-ny, boo-boo! Nin-ny-nan-ny, noo-noo! Nin-ny-nan-ny, nin-ny-nan-ny, noo!

Oh, what a nin-ny! Oh, what a nan-ny!

Oh, what a nin-ny-nan-ny-noo! *(Chant)* Nin-ny-nan-ny, nin-ny-nan-ny,

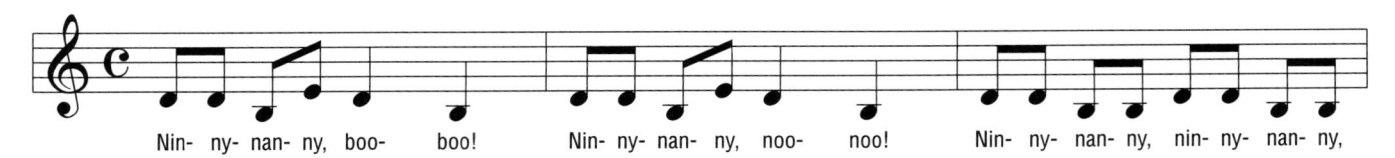

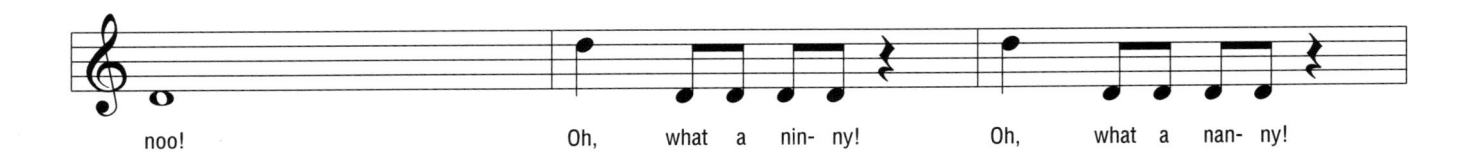

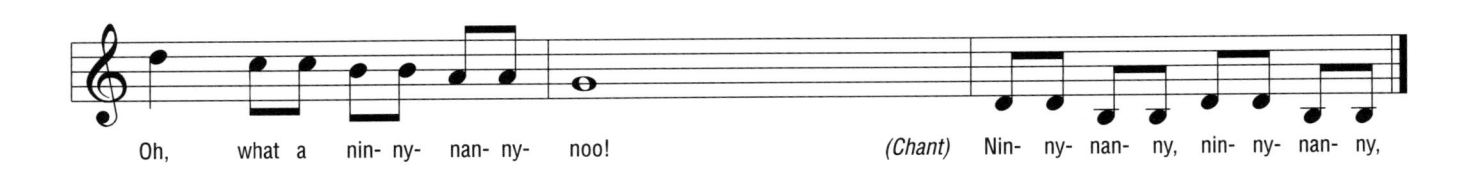

(Shout) **NOO!**

Purple Pipple Pop

Singing the Song

This song is sung as a group. Accent the "hiccup" with a sitting bounce in place.

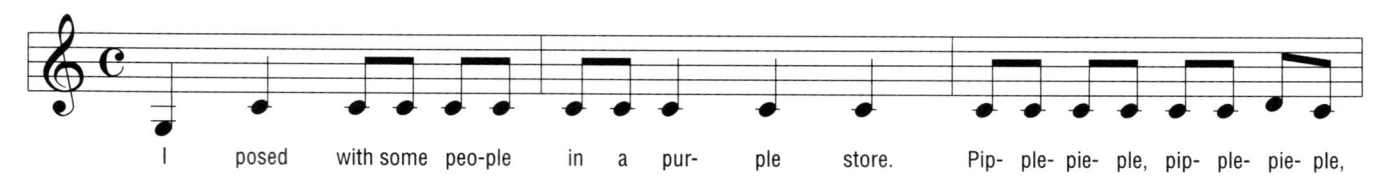

Purple Pipple Pop

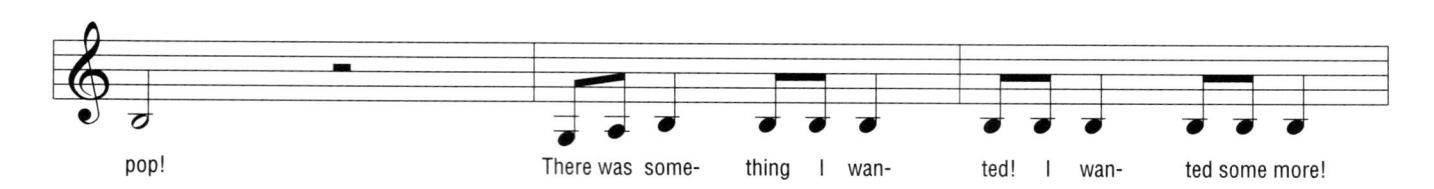

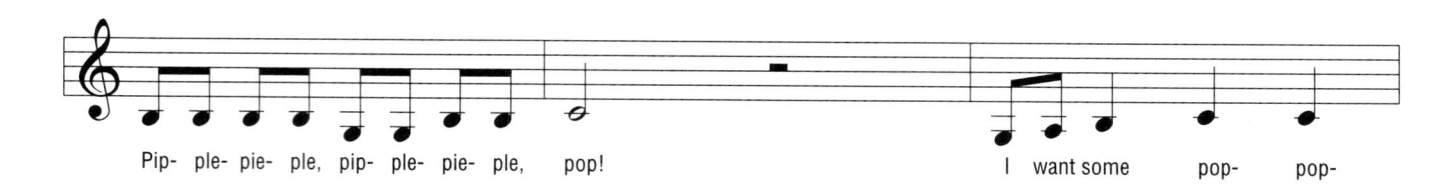

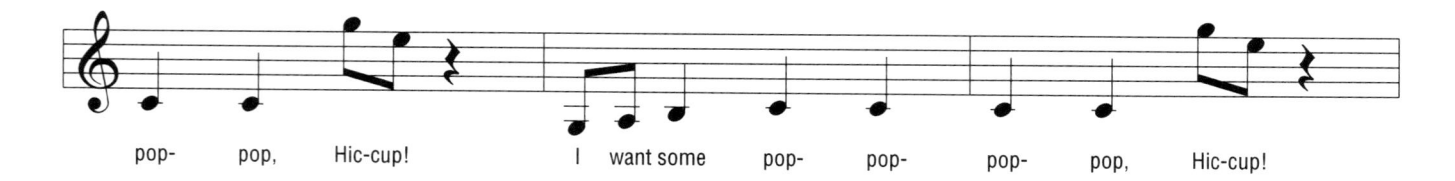

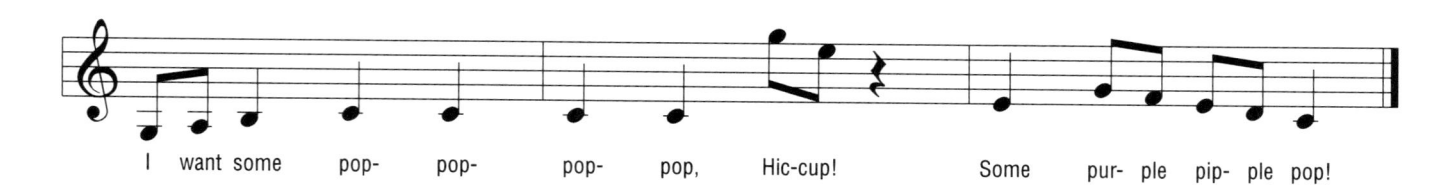

I posed with some peo-ple in a pur-ple store. Pip-ple-pie-ple, pip-ple-pie-ple, pop! There was some-thing I wan-ted! I wan-ted some more! Pip-ple-pie-ple, pip-ple-pie-ple, pop! I want some pop- pop- pop- pop, Hic-cup! I want some pop- pop- pop- pop, Hic-cup! I want some pop- pop- pop- pop, Hic-cup! Some pur-ple pip-ple pop!

Raving and Raring to Roar!

Playing the Game

Seat the children in a circle. Call one child to stand in the center of the circle. Ask the child to name a fierce animal. Substitute the name of the chosen animal for the word *lion*. Sing the verse lines, and have the children respond with the chorus lines. The child in the center pretends to be the ferocious animal and acts out the verse by pacing and making beastly faces. At the end of the song, the children stand up and roar together as one ferocious beast.

Raving and Raring to Roar!

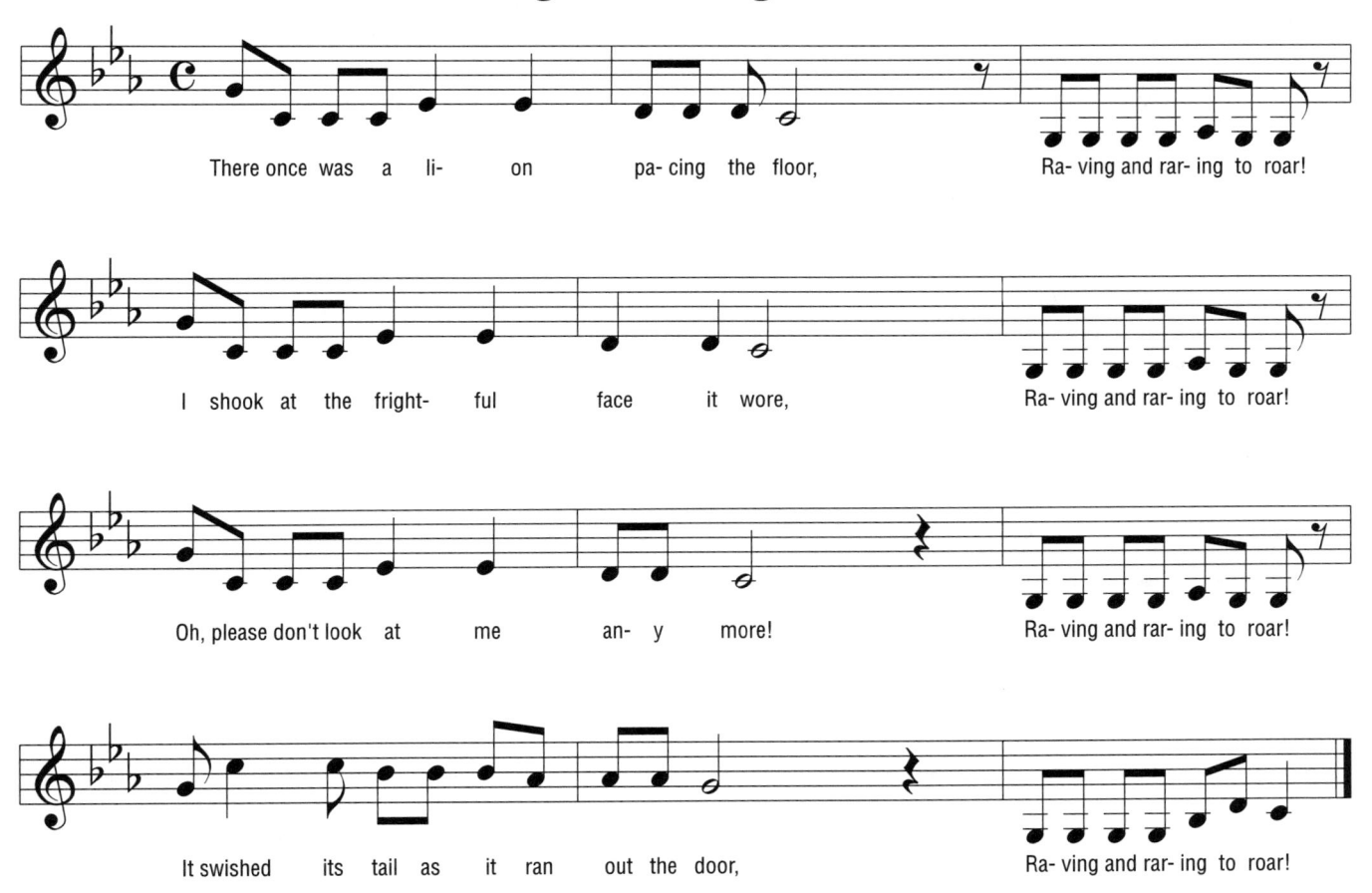

There once was a li- on pa- cing the floor, Ra- ving and rar- ing to roar!
I shook at the fright- ful face it wore, Ra- ving and rar- ing to roar!
Oh, please don't look at me an- y more! Ra- ving and rar- ing to roar!
It swished its tail as it ran out the door, Ra- ving and rar- ing to roar!

(Voiced) **Rrrrrr-RRRRRR-ROAR!**

Sally, the Silly Snake

Material

Two lengths of rope ("snakes"), each about one yard long

Playing the Game

Sit with the children in a circle. Divide the group into two teams around the circle; the children on your right are Team A, and the children on your left are Team B. (If there is an uneven number of children, name one child to be the scorekeeper for one round. At the end of the round, have that child join a group, and name another scorekeeper.) Hand one rope to the child on your right, and give the other rope to the child on your left. Those two children hold the ropes while all children sing the song. At the end of the verse, the children hiss and quickly pass the ropes around the circle in opposite directions. The object of the game is to be the first team to return one of the ropes to you. When the first rope reaches you, the round is over, the team on that side earns one point, and the "losing snake" is declared the "Silly Sally." Have the first pair of children move to the "halfway point" of the circle so that another pair of children moves to your right and left sides; and play another round. Play a predetermined number of rounds, or set a time limit, or play until interest wanes (or play until all children have had a turn being scorekeeper). The team with the most points wins the game.

Sally, the Silly Snake

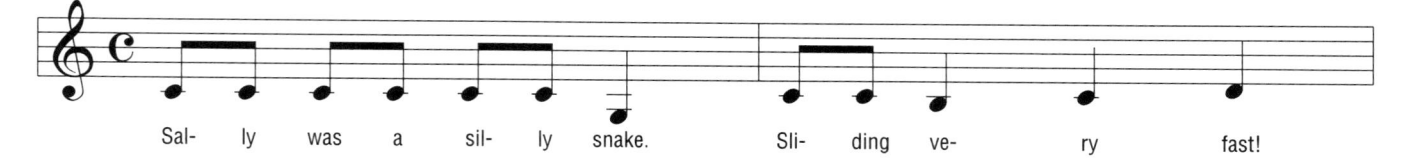

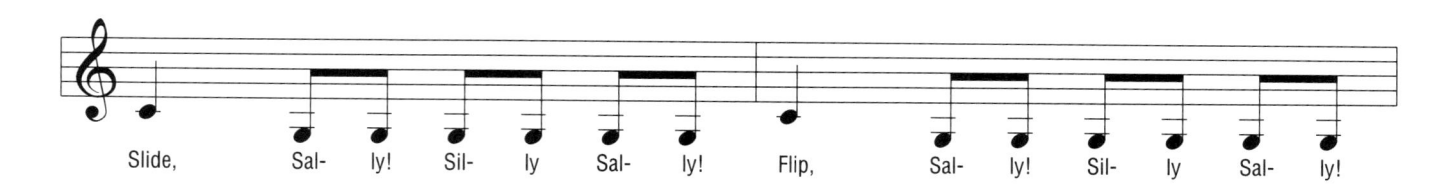

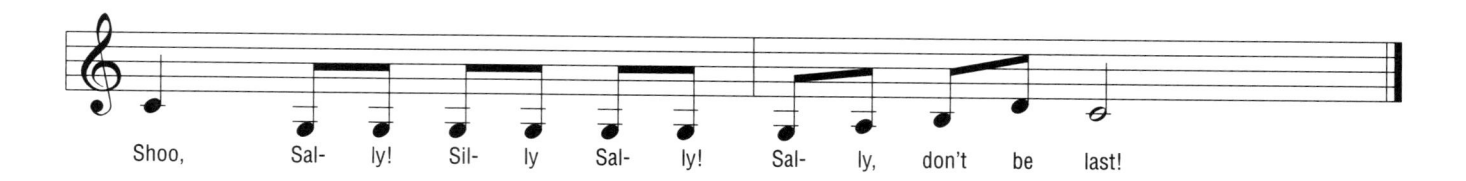

Sal-ly was a sil-ly snake. Sli-ding ve-ry fast!
Slide, Sal-ly! Sil-ly Sal-ly! Flip, Sal-ly! Sil-ly Sal-ly!
Shoo, Sal-ly! Sil-ly Sal-ly! Sal-ly, don't be last!

(Voiced) **HISSSS!**

Tippie-Tappie

Playing the Game

Seat the children on the floor. The song is sung in unison. On the words, "Tippie tappie talt," the group leans over to the left. On "tolt," the group leans to the right. When "tilt" is sung, the group leans forward; and on "spilt," all fall over backward.

Tippie-Tappie

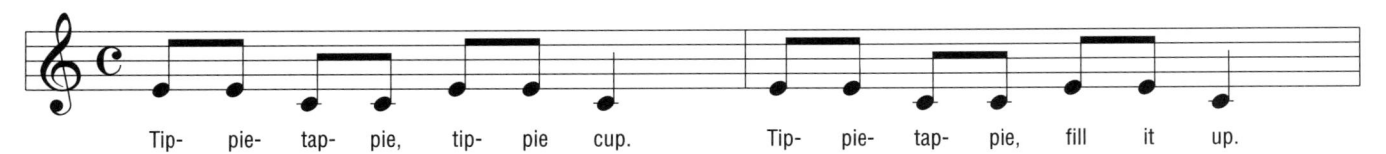

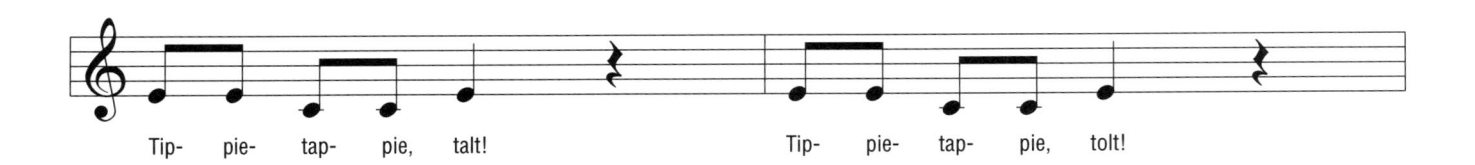

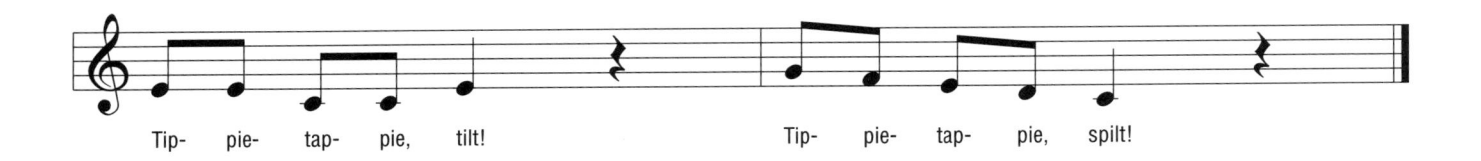

Tip- pie- tap- pie, tip- pie cup. Tip- pie- tap- pie, fill it up.

Tip- pie- tap- pie, talt! Tip- pie- tap- pie, tolt!

Tip- pie- tap- pie, tilt! Tip- pie- tap- pie, spilt!

Vittles in the Vat

Singing the Song

For each verse of this song, substitute a different vowel sound in the word "vittles."

Vittles in the Vat

Vit-tles in the vat! Vit-tles in the vat! Now, just who'd eat that? Vit-tles in the vat!
Vol-ly- vol-ly, vroom- vroom! Vit-tle- vit-tle, vit-tles in the vat!

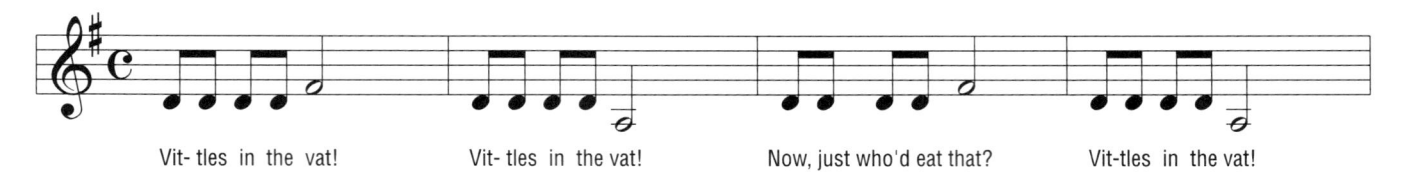

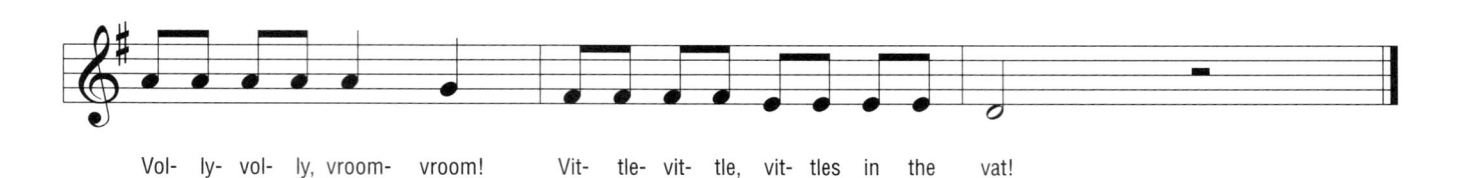

Verse 2: Vitals in the vat!
Verse 3: Vattles in the vat!
Verse 4: Veetles in the vat!
Verse 5: Vootles in the vat!

Wiggle-Wiggle, Whompa-Whompa, Woo!

Playing the Game

This is a counting song. As the group sings, "Wee wiggle one," all hold up the index finger on both hands. Move the index fingers next to the thumbs as the song directs. During the chorus, flex both index fingers back and forth as if they were puppets talking with each other. As the group sings, "Wee wiggle two," all hold up two fingers on both hands. The children move their fingers next to their shoes as the song directs. During the chorus, they flex the two fingers on each hand back and forth again as if they were puppets talking with each other. Repeat the actions for each verse, with a different number of fingers in a new place as indicated by the song.

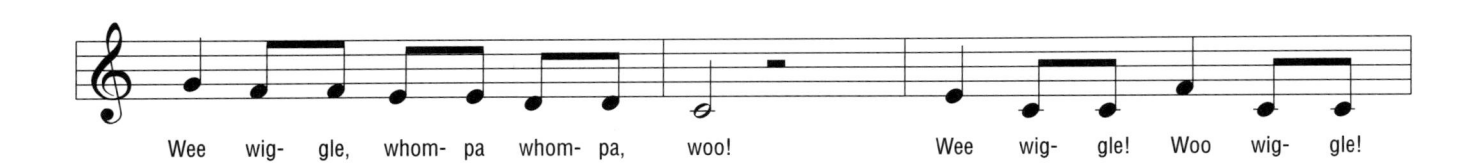

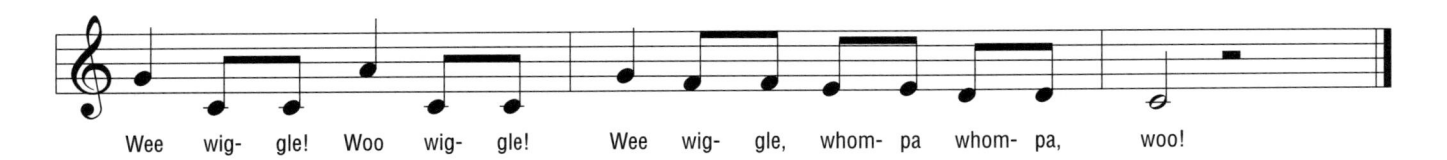

Wiggle-Wiggle, Whompa-Whompa, Woo!

Wee wig-gle one, Next to my thumb.
Wee wig-gle, whom-pa whom-pa, woo! Wee wig-gle! Woo wig-gle!
Wee wig-gle! Woo wig-gle! Wee wig-gle, whom-pa whom-pa, woo!

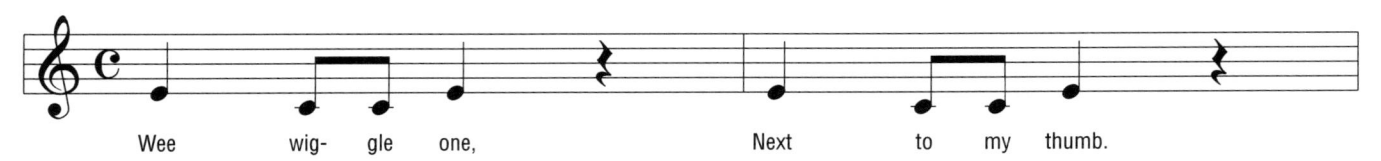

(Shout) WOO!

Verse 2:
Wee wiggle two, Next to my shoe.
Wee wiggle, whompa whompa, woo!

Verse 3:
Wee wiggle three, Next to my knee.
Wee wiggle, whompa whompa, woo!

Verse 4:
Wee wiggle four, Next to the floor.
Wee wiggle, whompa whompa, woo!

Verse 5:
Wee wiggle five, Wiggle wag alive!
Wee wiggle, whompa whompa, woo!

Yippee! Yappie! Ki-Yi-Yay!

Playing the Game

The children stand in a circle. Ask the children to join hands and then release them once the circle is obtained. For children who will not stay in one place, the hands may remain joined until the chorus. Sing the lines and have the children respond with "Yippie! Yappie! Ki-yi-yay!" On the chorus, all sing and walk or run in a circle, pretending to ride horses.

Yippee! Yappie! Ki-Yi-Yay!

What does the cow-boy say? Yip-pie! Yap-pie! Ki-yi-yay! What does he do all day?

Yip-pie! Yap-pie! Ki-yi-yay! Does he ride his horse all day? Yip-pie! Yap-pie! Ki-yi-yay!

Ro-ping dog-ies as they play. Yip-pie! Yap-pie! Ki-yi-yay! Yip-pie-ki! Yip-pie-ki!

Yip-pie! Yap-pie! Ki-yi-yay! Yip-pie-ki! Yip-pie-ki! Yip-pie! Yap-pie! Ki-yi-yay!

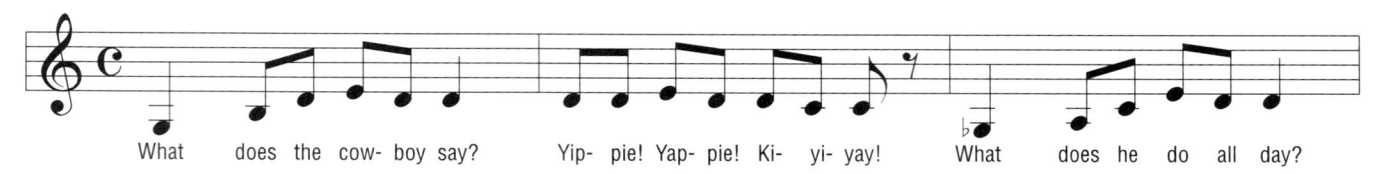

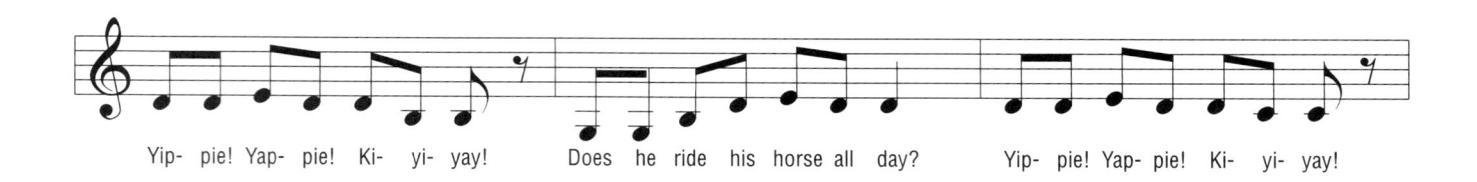

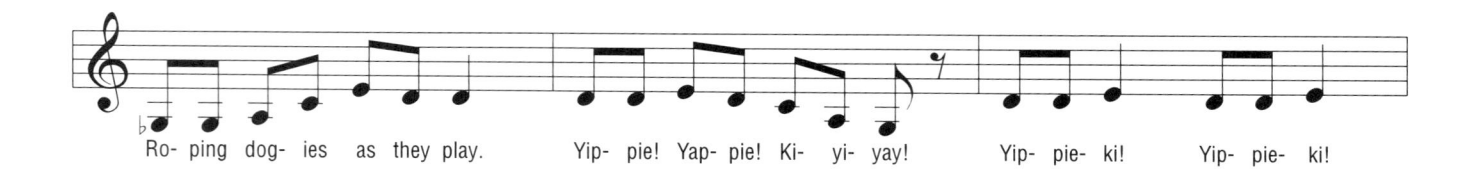

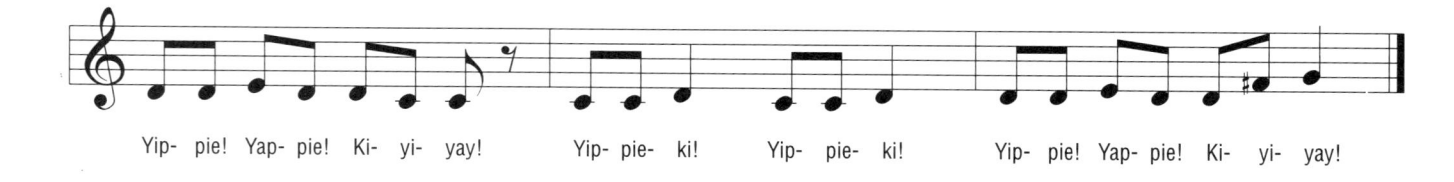

(Shout) **YEE HAW!**

Zap!

After the verses are sung, repeat this tune making a continuous "ZZZZZZZ" sound. End the song with a shouted "Zap!"

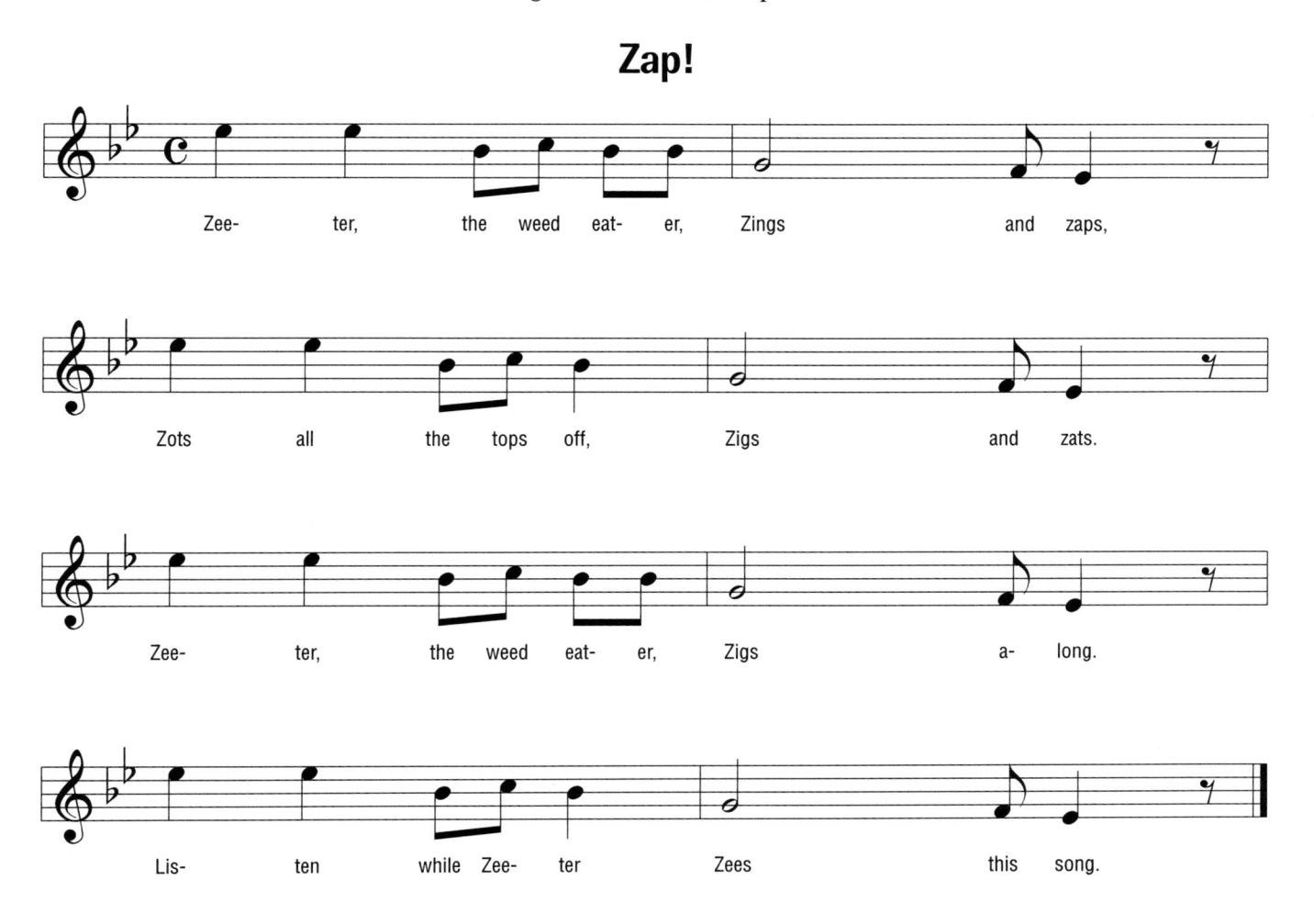

Zap!

Zee- ter, the weed eat- er, Zings and zaps,

Zots all the tops off, Zigs and zats.

Zee- ter, the weed eat- er, Zigs a- long.

Lis- ten while Zee- ter Zees this song.

Repeat the tune, making a continuous ZZZZZZZ sound.

(Shout) **ZAP!**